COPING WITH CHEMOTHERAPY

TERRY PRIESTMAN is consultant clinical oncologist working at New Cross Hospital, Wolverhampton. He is also medical reviewer for the charity CancerBACUP (which provides information for cancer patients, their relatives and health professionals). He has written more than a hundred papers in the medical press, and is a past Dean of the faculty of Clinical Oncology at the Royal College of Radiologists.

Overcoming Common Problems Series

Selected titles
A full list of titles is available from Sheldon Press,
36 Causton Street, London SW1P 4ST, and on our website at
www.sheldonpress.co.uk

Overcoming Common Problems Series

Overcoming Common Problems Series

Overcoming Common Problems

Coping with Chemotherapy

Dr Terry Priestman

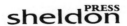

First published in Great Britain in 2005

Sheldon Press
36 Causton Street
London SW1P 4ST

Copyright © Terry Priestman 2005

British Library Cataloguing-in-Publication Data

A catalogue record for this book is available from the British Library

ISBN 0–85969–949–8

1 3 5 7 9 10 8 6 4 2

Typeset by Deltatype Limited, Birkenhead, Merseyside
Printed in Great Britain by
Ashford Colour Press

Contents

To everyone, past and present, who has been associated with the Deanesley Centre, New Cross Hospital, Wolverhampton

Introduction

Every year in the UK nearly 200,000 people discover they have cancer. Overall, about one in three of us can expect to develop cancer at some time during our lives. The good news to set against these depressing figures, though, is that over the last 30 years the outlook for people with most types of cancer has greatly improved. Complete cures are now possible for many cancers; and even when the condition is incurable, treatment can often offer many years of good-quality life before the illness reaches its terminal stage.

Chemotherapy plays a major part in cancer treatment, and has transformed the outlook for many types of cancer over the last few decades. Very often, cures are now possible that could never have been imagined in the 1950s and 1960s. These days at least half of all people who are diagnosed with cancer are likely to have some form of chemotherapy, at some time, during their illness.

Although it has led to a big rise in the number of people being permanently cured, and considerable increases in life expectancy for many other people where cure was not possible, chemotherapy is still a word that usually causes great anxiety and distress when it is first mentioned as being part of someone's treatment. To most people it means months of upsetting side effects, with a devastating impact on their day-to-day lives. But although it can be very traumatic and disruptive, many people find that when they actually get started on treatment it is not nearly as bad as they had expected, and they are able to cope with it remarkably well. Very often the reality of chemotherapy is far less unpleasant than people imagine.

Much of the fear about chemotherapy comes from not really knowing what to expect, or what will happen, or what to do when things do happen. These days, if you are going to have chemotherapy, you are likely to be given lots of information about your treatment. But often this is passed on verbally by doctors or nurses in busy clinics where it is difficult to take in, and it can also be hard to ask questions if there are things you don't understand. Even if you are given leaflets or booklets to back up what has been said at the hospital, these may only cover some aspects of your treatment, or be written in a way that is difficult to make sense of – or you may feel it just doesn't apply to you.

The aim of this book is to try to fill in the background about what chemotherapy is, what it does, and how to carry on with life during, and after, your treatment. As the book is designed to cover the whole subject, only bits of it are likely to apply to your own situation, so it is probably something you will find more helpful to dip into and out of, rather than to read from cover to cover. It is not intended to replace information that you may be given at hospital, but to be used alongside it – perhaps to fill in some gaps, or to give additional reassurance, or help you understand things by having them explained in a slightly different way.

Many people say that being aware of what is going on, understanding what to expect, and knowing what to do when and if problems crop up, makes coping with their treatment much easier. Being informed can greatly reduce the anxieties and uncertainties of chemotherapy, and can give you more control over what is happening to you.

1

What is chemotherapy?

The word 'chemotherapy' was first used by doctors to describe the use of drugs, like antibiotics, that were given to treat infections. When, about 60 years ago, the first drugs were discovered that could be given to treat cancer, the term was extended to include the use of these new compounds. In recent years, people have become much more aware of drug treatment for cancer – partly because of its considerable success in increasing the number of cures, which means that more people than ever are having the treatment, and partly because of the sometimes distressing side effects that it can cause. With this growing public awareness, the word 'chemotherapy' has increasingly come to be shorthand for 'cancer chemotherapy' and its original, broader meaning has largely been lost.

What is cancer?

Before going any further, it is important to be clear what we mean by the word 'cancer'.

We all begin our lives as a single cell fertilized in our mother's womb. That cell then divides to form two cells, those two cells divide to make four, and this process of cell division continues throughout pregnancy, and on through infancy, childhood and adolescence, to produce the countless billions of cells that make up our adult selves.

Even in adulthood the process of cell growth continues, because cells are constantly wearing out and dying off and need to be replaced. For example, the bone marrow, which produces the red cells, white cells and platelets that make up our blood, makes many millions of new cells every day to replace those that have worn out. Similarly, the cells that line parts of our digestive system are replaced every 24–48 hours.

Throughout our lives, these processes of cell division and growth are very precisely controlled so that we make exactly the number of new cells that our bodies need – no more, no less.

A cancer develops when the cells in a particular organ escape from these controls and begin to reproduce and grow in a haphazard way, producing more cells than they should. Over time, these cells build up to form a tumour, or growth. If this is not treated, then the growth will begin to invade and destroy the tissue surrounding it. It may also send off seedlings – tiny clumps of cells – that spread to form secondary growths in other parts of the body. These seedlings may be carried either in the bloodstream, or through the lymph vessels – the network of threadlike channels that drain fluid from the tissues into the lymph glands (lymph nodes).

Tumours can be divided into two main types: benign and malignant. Benign tumours may grow to a large size, but they do not actually invade and destroy the tissue surrounding them, and they do not spread to other parts of the body. Malignant tumours are able both to invade and destroy nearby tissue, and to form secondary growths. The word 'cancer' only applies to these growths; a benign tumour is not a cancer, but a malignant tumour is.

Most cancers start as a single growth in one part of the body; this is called the primary cancer. As it continues to grow, the primary cancer may, or may not, produce secondary cancers elsewhere. Another name for these secondary cancers is metastases. When a doctor or nurse talks about metastatic cancer, they mean a cancer that has already spread to other parts of the body.

Types of chemotherapy

There are several different types of drug treatment that can be used to treat cancer.

The first of these to be developed is known as cytotoxic chemotherapy. Cytotoxic drugs are, as their name suggests, cell poisons. They work by damaging the cancer cell so that it is unable to divide, and reproduce, and therefore it dies. Today there are more than 100 different cytotoxic drugs that can be used in the treatment of cancer. Unfortunately, none of these drugs is able to tell the difference between cancer cells and normal cells. This means that when these drugs are given, they will cause some damage to normal cells as well as killing off the cancer cells, and this is why they can cause side effects.

The great majority of people who have drugs as part of their cancer treatment will be given cytotoxics. Because of this, when we talk about chemotherapy today, what we usually mean is cytotoxic chemotherapy.

Another type of drug treatment for cancer, developed at about the same time as cytotoxic drugs first appeared, is hormone treatment. Hormone therapy is only suitable for a very few types of cancer, but it does play an important part in the treatment of two very common conditions: breast cancer and prostate cancer. Hormonal drugs work very differently to cytotoxics, and generally cause fewer side effects.

More recently, other types of compounds have been discovered that can help in cancer treatment. These include agents such as interferons, and monoclonal antibodies, which are often given along with cytotoxic drugs to increase their effectiveness.

But because cytotoxic chemotherapy accounts for the majority of the drug-based cancer treatments, and because it is what most people mean when they use the word 'chemotherapy', the rest of this book will deal mainly with cytotoxic drugs rather than other types of therapy.

Chemotherapy and radiotherapy

Chemotherapy and radiotherapy are both important types of cancer treatment. People sometimes confuse them, but they are very different. Chemotherapy relies on drugs, whereas radiotherapy uses high-energy, ionising radiation to kill cancer cells.

Most radiotherapy treatments are given using machines called linear accelerators (or LinAcs, for short). The LinAc produces a beam of very high-energy x-rays that can be focused on the part of the body where the cancer is. The patient lies on a couch by the machine for a few minutes for each treatment. The treatment itself is completely painless. Depending on the type of cancer, and the reason for the treatment, a course of radiotherapy can last anywhere from a single dose to 30–40 doses over 6–8 weeks.

An important difference between radiotherapy and chemotherapy is that radiotherapy is a localized treatment. That is, it is only given to a particular part of the body where the cancer is, or might be, present, and so it only affects that area. With chemotherapy, the drugs that are used pass into the bloodstream and will reach almost all parts of the body, so it is a general treatment – or, to use the medical word, a systemic treatment.

How did it all begin?

Modern-day cancer chemotherapy has its origins in the Second World War. During the Italian campaign, in late 1943, a convoy of Allied ships was moored in the harbour at Bari. Unexpectedly, the Luftwaffe launched one of their last major raids of the war and a number of the ships were hit, and exploded. Inevitably there were casualties, but a few days after the attack people in the port area became unwell, with signs of skin damage and infection. Many were admitted to hospital and, despite the best efforts of the medical staff, died from their mysterious illness. Among the doctors involved at the time were two American army physicians, who noted that nearly all their patients had very low white blood cell counts, lowering their resistance to infection.

Although it was kept a closely guarded secret at the time, it was later revealed to the doctors that one of the ships at Bari had a cargo of shells containing the poison gas mustine, or nitrogen mustard. These shells had exploded and released a cloud of the gas over the harbour area, and this was the cause of the previously unexplained deaths.

Thinking about the tragedy later, the American doctors realized that although the effect of the nitrogen mustard on the Bari patients' white blood cells had been disastrous, there were illnesses where such an effect might actually be beneficial. Leukaemias and lymphomas are types of cancer where the main problem is an over-production of white blood cells. Doctors reasoned that if they could inject people who had leukaemia and lymphoma with small doses of nitrogen mustard, then it might lower their numbers of white blood cells and help to control their illness.

Back in the USA, they tried some experiments on volunteers with these cancers, and discovered that, for a time at least, they could improve their condition. So nitrogen mustard suddenly transformed from an agent of biological warfare to the first anti-cancer drug, and ushered in the age of cancer chemotherapy.

Since the late 1940s the story of chemotherapy has two main threads: the discovery of new drugs, and working out how best to use them.

The discovery of new drugs

The realization that nitrogen mustard could help to control some types of leukaemia and lymphoma opened the floodgates for research to find other drugs that might be more effective, and that might have fewer side effects (because nitrogen mustard was quite a toxic treatment).

To begin with, the work centred around looking at compounds that were chemically similar to mustine. Within a few years, this led to the development of drugs like cyclophosphamide and chlorambucil, which are still widely used today.

Other families of chemicals were soon discovered which, although still attacking the process of cell division and multiplication, worked in different ways to nitrogen mustard and its successors. These included synthetic compounds, like methotrexate and fluorouracil, and natural preparations like the Vinca alkaloids (extracts of the periwinkle plant Vinca rosea), vincristine and vinblastine. Although over 50 years old, all these drugs still have an important role in cancer treatment in the twenty-first century.

Since the 1950s, many other compounds with anti-cancer activity have been introduced so that we now have more than 100 different drugs available. The great majority of these, like the early drugs, are cytotoxic agents, and stop cells reproducing. In more recent years, however, there has been a lot of interest in developing drugs that specifically target cancer cells – unlike the cytotoxics, which affect normal and malignant tissues. The most important group of drugs here are the monoclonal antibodies. These have only been appearing in the last few years, and at the present time they are mainly given along with cytotoxics rather than being used as an alternative to them, but as more and better types of these drugs are discovered, that could well change.

If we have so many drugs that attack cancer, why hasn't everyone been cured and why are we still looking for new drugs? The first thing to say is that for many types of cancer the outlook has been transformed by the developments in chemotherapy over the last 50 years. Many conditions that in the 1950s and 1960s were usually fatal can now be almost always cured.

But unfortunately this isn't universally true, and some cancers do remain a challenge. This is partly because various types of cancer respond differently to the drugs we have available – a treatment that works very well in one tumour type will often be completely ineffective in another. It is also the case that in some growths, which seem at first to be responsive to the treatment, resistant cancer cells will develop that are immune to the effects of chemotherapy and will continue to grow and cause problems.

So we are still looking for the 'miracle cure', the 'wonder drug', the 'magic bullet', that will provide the final answer for cancer treatment. The search goes on, and new drugs are being discovered all the time. But, in parallel with this process of drug development, a better understanding of how to use the treatments we already have has also helped to improve results over the years.

How we use chemotherapy

When the first cytotoxic drugs appeared in the 1940s they were a completely novel form of treatment, and no one was sure how to use them.

At first doctors turned to the principles of antibiotic therapy as a guide, which had been established a few years before. These suggested that just a single drug should be used, and it should be given sufficiently often to keep a fairly constant level of the drug in the blood at all times. With cytotoxics, the actual dose of the drug given was limited by its side effects, and was adjusted to stop these becoming too troublesome. This practice of giving one drug on a regular basis was called 'single agent continuous therapy'. Single agent continuous therapy did have some limited success in the 1950s, producing temporary improvements (but only temporary) in some advanced cancers, and actually leading to cures in two rare forms of cancer, Burkitt's lymphoma (an uncommon type of cancer of the lymph glands) and choriocarcinoma (a cancer affecting the womb, which occurs as a very rare complication of pregnancy). But in the common cancers, this new drug treatment had very little impact.

By the 1960s, with more drugs available, doctors realized that various cytotoxics could affect the process of cell division in different ways. This led to the idea of giving two or more drugs at the same time, in the hope that by combining their different modes of action they would increase the number of cancer cells killed. This multiple drug continuous therapy was used only briefly because it was rapidly found that, although it did increase the damage to some cancers, it had a dramatic effect on the toxicity of treatment, causing very severe, sometimes lethal, side effects.

The breakthrough in overcoming this problem was the realization that normal cells were much better, and much quicker, at repairing the damage caused by chemotherapy drugs than cancer cells. This led to the suggestion, in the late 1960s, that it would be better to give the drugs as intermittent courses, or cycles, with a rest interval with no treatment in between, rather than giving them continuously. The idea was that during the rest interval between courses, the normal cells would be able to recover completely from any damage caused by the drugs, while the cancer cells would still not have made good the harmful effects of the previous course. The next course would then damage the cancer cells still further. In this way, a number of courses could be given, with normal cells bouncing back between each cycle, while cancer cells were progressively killed off until they had disappeared completely. This was called 'intermittent combination chemotherapy'.

Intermittent combination chemotherapy revolutionized cancer treatment, and has led to dramatic improvements in cure rates, or increased survival times, in many types of cancer since the 1970s. It is still the principle underpinning the use of cytotoxic chemotherapy today.

The other main development that occurred during the 1970s and 1980s was the use of drug treatment in the early stages of the disease. Up until then, chemotherapy had usually only been given to people with advanced cancer, which had spread widely through the body. Very occasionally, in a few types of cancer, this could bring about a cure, but usually all that happened was that the growth would shrink, or possibly even disappear, for a time, but then would start growing again and still be ultimately incurable.

It was then suggested that in some types of cancer there might be a benefit in giving chemotherapy much earlier, immediately after initial surgical treatment to remove the primary tumour – the hope being that this would prevent secondary cancers developing in the first place, rather than waiting for them to appear before starting the drugs. This idea of giving chemotherapy as an insurance policy to protect someone against the cancer coming back is called 'adjuvant therapy'. The introduction of adjuvant chemotherapy has increased cure rates in a number of major cancers over the last 20 years, including breast cancer and bowel cancer.

2

Who needs chemotherapy?

Some basic facts about cancer

Between one in three and one in four of us will develop a cancer at some time during our lives. There are more than 200 different types of cancer that can affect our bodies. Some cancers are very common, while others are very uncommon. For example, each year in Britain about 40,000 people are diagnosed with lung cancer, but cancer of the heart is virtually unknown; similarly, while there are about 35,000 new cases of cancer of the large bowel (the colon and rectum) each year, only a handful of cancers of the small bowel are discovered. Some cancers grow very rapidly – certain forms of acute leukaemia and some types of lung cancer can be fatal within a few weeks if they are not treated – whereas others progress extremely slowly; some chronic leukaemias, and prostate cancer in older men, can often go for years without needing treatment or causing any problems.

Some cancers, like breast cancers and cancers of the kidney, have a strong tendency to spread to other parts of the body, while others, like rodent ulcers of the skin, hardly ever give rise to secondary cancers. Some cancers cause symptoms, and are diagnosed at a very early stage in their development – for example, cancers of the vocal cord, which cause hoarseness of the voice – but others often only cause problems when they have reached a more advanced stage, and so are diagnosed much later in their development; this is often the case with cancers of the pancreas and the ovary.

About four out of every five cancers develop in cells that form the lining of the various organs of our bodies. These cells are called epithelial cells, and a cancer of the epithelial cells is called a carcinoma. So a carcinoma of the stomach is a cancer of the epithelial cells that form the inner lining of the stomach. Cancers of the supportive tissues of our bodies, the bones, muscles, fatty tissue and cartilage, are much less common, making up less than one in twenty cancers. These cancers of supportive tissue are called sarcomas. So a sarcoma of the stomach is a cancer of the muscular wall of that organ.

Both carcinomas and sarcomas typically begin as a single growth, the primary cancer, in a single organ, which may then spread to form secondary cancers in other parts of the body at a later time. By contrast, the other two major groups of cancers, the lymphomas and leukaemias, which make up about one in eight cancers, usually affect multiple sites throughout the body from their outset.

Lymphomas are cancers that arise in the lymph nodes, or in patches of lymphatic tissue which can be found in many of our body's organs. Leukaemias develop in the bone marrow and can also affect the lymph nodes and other organs.

Clearly, then, cancers make up a very diverse group of illnesses, and therefore very different approaches to treatment are needed for the various types of cancer.

Cancer treatment

With such a spectrum of diseases, the treatment that is needed varies enormously depending on the particular type of cancer. In broad terms, there are three main approaches to treatment: surgery, radiotherapy and drugs.

Surgery remains the cornerstone of treatment for most cancers, and still accounts for the majority of cures. When dealing with carcinomas and sarcomas, provided that the primary growth has not become too large, or spread to form metastases in other places, then an operation to remove the growth has a good chance of curing the condition. Although surgery is very often curative, it may fail for one of two reasons: either because microscopic traces of tumour, which would have been invisible to the surgeon, have been left behind, or because, again at a level too small to be detected, minute seedlings of the growth have already spread to form secondary cancers elsewhere.

Radiotherapy is often given after surgery to guard against the possibility of traces of cancer being left behind at the site of the operation. For example, in breast cancer, removing the primary tumour, either with a mastectomy, which takes the whole breast away, or a more conservative operation like a lumpectomy or wide local excision, apparently gets rid of the primary tumour. But if nothing more is done, then in about three out of ten people, in the months or years after surgery, microscopic remnants of the cancer that were missed will grow to form a local recurrence of the disease. Giving radiotherapy to the area after surgery is a way of reducing this risk, and lowers the level of local recurrences very dramatically. Radiotherapy is very often used in this way, as an adjunct to surgery, to reduce the risk of the tumour coming back.

One advantage of radiotherapy is that it can safely cover a wider volume of tissue than can be removed at an operation, and so can include the microscopic strands of cancer that may have infiltrated the normal tissue surrounding the primary growth, which would have been invisible at the time of the operation. In other situations, radiotherapy may actually be used as an alternative to surgery as a curative treatment in its own right. It also has an important role in the more advanced stages of many cancers, when it can help in easing distressing symptoms like pain, bleeding and breathlessness.

Although drug treatment has always been the mainstay of therapy for cancers like lymphomas and leukaemias (and often results in a cure), for many years chemotherapy was only used in the treatment of the more advanced stages of carcinomas and sarcomas. Here it often was, and still is, successful in shrinking the disease, sometimes even making it disappear for a while, and increasing life expectancy, but almost inevitably the cancer would come back at some future time. In more recent years it has been used increasingly in the earlier stages of cancer, alongside surgery and/or radiotherapy, increasing the chances of a cure. This latter approach is known as adjuvant chemotherapy, and because many people find it rather difficult to understand, it is worth a little more explanation.

Adjuvant chemotherapy

Adjuvant chemotherapy has been most widely used in breast cancer, and using this condition as an example is probably the easiest way to explain how it works.

Although surgery and radiotherapy will cure many women of their breast cancers, some women who appear to have been cured will need further treatment, months or years later, with signs of spread of the disease to other parts of the body, such as the bones, liver, lungs or brain. These secondary cancers must have been present, as microscopic, undetectable, seedlings of tumour, before the primary cancer was removed. The primary cancer could not have sent off

10

metastases to other parts of the body after it had been taken away. The fact that these minute secondaries were missed when the original treatment was carried out was not a mistake by the doctors at the time: it was simply that whatever examinations, blood tests, x-rays or scans had been done, the tumours would have been too small to show up.

By the early 1970s the introduction of intermittent combination cytotoxic chemotherapy, giving three or more drugs together in cycles, or pulses, with rest periods in between to allow normal tissues to recover, had proved very effective in the more advanced stages of breast cancer, when the disease was extensive and incurable. The drugs would often reduce the size and number of the secondary cancers, relieve unpleasant symptoms and regularly extend survival, although they would not bring about a permanent cure. At the same time a new hormonal drug, tamoxifen, was discovered, which also helped in controlling advanced breast cancer.

As a result of these developments in treatment, doctors began to wonder if giving cytotoxic chemotherapy, or tamoxifen, or both, to women who had apparently been cured by surgery and radiotherapy might completely kill off any microscopic seedlings of tumour that had spread elsewhere, and so increase these women's chances of a long-term cure.

In theory this was a good idea, but one problem was that not everyone who had surgery and radiotherapy for their early breast cancer would need the drugs. Some women would have been truly cured by their original treatment, while others would only appear to have been cured, and would still be at risk. But as the secondary cancers that posed that risk were too small to be detected, how could doctors know which women did, or did not, need the drugs?

The answer was to find some feature of the cancer that suggested that a woman might be more at risk of harbouring those tiny seedlings of tumour spread. Doctors turned to statistics that suggested that if the results of the initial surgery showed that the cancer had spread to one or more of the nearby lymph glands under the arm, on the same side as the affected breast, then even if those nodes were removed completely, there was a greater likelihood that undetectable secondaries would be present in other sites than if the glands had all been completely free of tumour.

In the mid-1970s clinical trials began whereby women who had surgery to remove their breast cancer, but who were found to have one or more nearby lymph nodes involved with the cancer, were either given chemotherapy, or tamoxifen, or both, or no further treatment. It soon became apparent that the women who received the drug therapy had a much better chance of cure, and giving the additional treatment rapidly became standard practice.

Since then, trials have continued, and are still ongoing, to work out as precisely as possible who actually needs the treatment, and what is the best combination of drugs for each individual patient.

Over time, this principle of adjuvant, or precautionary, chemotherapy has also been extended to other types of cancer; it has proved valuable in bowel cancer, ovarian cancer and a number of other tumour types. Incidentally, although adjuvant chemotherapy is usually given after surgery, it is occasionally used before an operation is carried out; this is then referred to as neo-adjuvant therapy.

Although it can greatly improve someone's chance of a cure with certain types of cancer, there are at least two aspects of this adjuvant therapy that people often find hard to understand. The first is that, having had their initial surgery and/or radiotherapy, many people feel completely well and, as they have no apparent signs or symptoms of cancer, find it difficult to accept that they may need extra treatment, which can often go on for many months, and may cause troublesome side effects. Furthermore, even when all that treatment is complete, there is no way of telling if it has been successful. Since there was no detectable or measurable cancer remaining in the first place, there is no test that can be done at the end of the treatment to see if those microscopic remnants of the disease, which may or may not have been present, have been destroyed. Unfortunately, some people may need to wait several months or even years to ascertain whether the cancer has been completely cleared from their bodies.

So who needs chemotherapy?

For many people with cancer, surgery or radiotherapy, or a combination of the two, will result in a cure and they will not need any further treatment. But chemotherapy may be needed in the following situations:

- It may be the best first line of treatment to cure or control certain types of cancer. This is most likely to be the case in cancers like lymphomas and leukaemias.

- It may be a wise precaution following surgery and/or radiotherapy in certain types of cancer to maximize the chances of cure, and minimize the risk of the cancer coming back (adjuvant treatment).
- It may be given in the more advanced stages of some cancers, occasionally in the hope of achieving a cure, but more often with the intention of controlling the disease, relieving symptoms, and increasing life expectancy.
- It may be used to shrink the size of a cancer before surgery or radiotherapy is given (neo-adjuvant therapy).

3

Which drugs are used?

In the 60 years since the first anti-cancer drug, nitrogen mustard, was discovered, more than 100 different cytotoxic agents have been used in cancer treatment. Some are much more widely used than others, and this chapter will mention a few of the most important compounds. There is also a short explanation of how hormonal drugs and new agents work in order to show how these differ from cytotoxic drugs.

The cytotoxic drugs have been grouped together in different families, based on their different ways of interfering with the process of cell division. Before describing these, a few words about the way in which cells divide might be helpful.

Cell division

Both normal cells and cancer cells are made up of a nucleus surrounded by a layer of cytoplasm. The nucleus contains the genetic material that determines how that cell will behave. This genetic information is carried in the genes. The genes are made up of a protein called DNA, and the DNA is made up of two strands of chemicals, twisted around one another in a spiral.

These genes are strung out along the chromosomes, a bit like pearls on a necklace. Each nucleus contains 23 pairs of these chromosomes. When the cell is getting ready to reproduce, and divide in two, it makes sufficient new DNA to form a complete new set of genes, and chromosomes.

At the beginning of cell division the two DNA strands making up each of the genes separate, and act as templates to form new matching strands, made up from the DNA in the nucleus. This means that two new genes are created, and their genetic information will be exactly the same as the original ones, ensuring that the two new cells that will be produced retain the characteristics of the parent cell.

These new genes will then make up two new sets of chromosomes. When these have been completed, the wall of the nucleus dissolves and the two sets of chromosomes separate to opposite sides

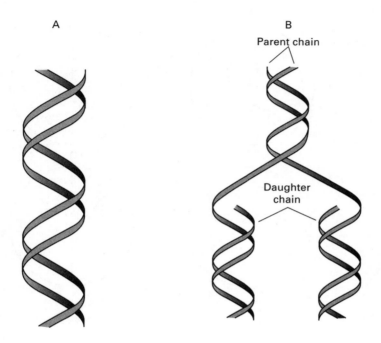

Figure 1 Cell division: DNA replication

A   The normal DNA, which makes up our genes, is in the cell nucleus, and is made up of two strands of chemicals coiled around one another.

B   The first stage of cell division is for these strands to separate and form templates for the creation of daughter strands, so that two new sets of DNA are formed, which are identical to the original, parent DNA.

15

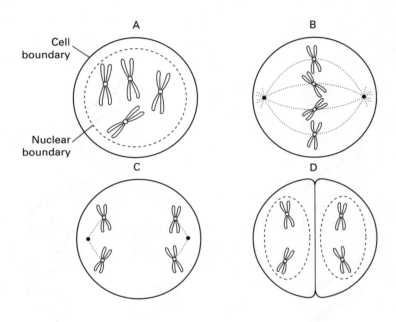

Figure 2 Cell division: mitosis

A   The two new sets of DNA are used to build two sets of genes and chromosomes in the nucleus (prophase)

B   The two new sets of chromosomes become arranged along the thread-like cell spindle (metaphase)

C   The chromosomes move along the spindle to opposite sides of the nucleus, and the spindle begins to disappear (anaphase)

D   The nucleus divides in two, each new nucleus now containing a complete set of chromosomes, identical to those in the original cell (telophase)

16

of the cell, moving along a grid of fine tubes called the cell spindle. Once the separation of the two sets of chromosomes is complete, the cytoplasm divides around them and the two new cells are created.

This process of cell division is called mitosis.

The major families of cytotoxic drugs

Before describing these, a few words of explanation about drug names might be a good idea. Rather confusingly, most drugs in the UK have two names, a non-proprietary (proper) name, and a proprietary (brand) name. The non-proprietary name is the scientific name of the particular compound. The proprietary name is the trade name of the drug, which has been patented by the company that makes it. Non-proprietary names are always written with the first letter in the lower case; for proprietary names, the first letter is always a capital. So, for example, Taxol is the trade name of the drug paclitaxel, and Campto is the trade name of the drug irinotecan. This means that during your treatment you might hear the same drug being talked about but with two different names. With older drugs, where the original manufacturer's patents have expired, often only the non-proprietary name is used. In this chapter, if a drug has a commonly used brand name it is given in brackets after its non-proprietary name.

Alkylating agents

The first cytotoxic to be discovered, nitrogen mustard, was an alkylating agent. It is little used nowadays, but a number of related compounds are still important. Two of these are cyclophosphamide, which is used to treat many different cancers, including breast cancer and lung cancer, and chlorambucil, which is used for some lymphomas and some types of leukaemia.

The alkylating agents work by forming bonds between the two DNA strands so that when they try to separate, at the time of mitosis, they are broken up.

The anti-metabolites

These were the second group of anti-cancer drugs to be developed, and first began to appear in the late 1940s. Two of the oldest drugs, still in general use today, are methotrexate and fluorouracil. Both of

17

these are used to treat breast cancer. Fluorouracil is also used to treat cancer of the colon and rectum (cancer of the large bowel), and methotrexate is also used to treat cancer arising in the head and neck area. These days fluorouracil is usually given together with a vitamin, called leucovorin, which increases its effectiveness.

More recent anti-metabolites include gemcitabine (Gemzar), useful for cancer of the pancreas; fludarabine (Fludara), for use against some lymphomas; capecitabine (Xeloda), for cancer of the large bowel; and pemetrexed, for the asbestos-related cancer called mesothelioma.

The anti-metabolites all work by interfering with the production of new DNA, so that the cells are unable to make the material they need to produce new genes.

The anthracyclines

These are one group of a number of cytotoxic drugs that were developed from antibiotics. The two most important agents are epirubicin and doxorubicin. They are used in the treatment of breast cancer, lung cancer, stomach cancer and some lymphomas. They act by inserting themselves between the DNA strands, fitting rather like a key in a lock, and so wedging the strands together so that they cannot separate at the time of mitosis.

Other cytotoxic drugs derived from antibiotics include bleomycin, which is used to treat testicular cancer, and mitomycin, which is given for stomach cancer.

Platinum compounds

These are all based on the heavy metal, platinum. They were discovered by accident in the late 1960s when studies looking at the effect of electric currents on the growth of bacteria found that if probes made of platinum were used to supply the current, the bacteria died off. Further studies showed that, rather like the alkylating agents, platinum compounds can produce crosslinks between the DNA strands, stopping the reproduction process.

The three platinum compounds in common use today are cisplatin and carboplatin (Paraplatin), which are valuable in ovarian cancer, lung cancer, and testicular tumours, and more recently oxaliplatin (Eloxatin), which is used against cancers of the colon and rectum (bowel cancers).

Spindle poisons

These are drugs that interfere with a substance called tubulin, which is present in the cells. One of the things tubulin does is to make the cell spindle, which separates the new chromosomes during mitosis. So the damage to tubulin prevents the cell spindle from working properly and arrests the process of cell division.

The spindle cell poisons are all based on natural compounds. One group are the Vinca alkaloids, from the periwinkle plant Vinca rosea. These include vincristine (Oncovin) and vinblastine (Velbe), which are valuable in lymphoma treatment, and vinorelbine (Navelbine), which is used against breast and lung cancer. The second group are the taxanes, based on extracts from the bark of the Pacific yew tree. These are paclitaxel (Taxol) and docetaxol (Taxotere). They are used mainly against breast, ovarian and lung cancer.

Topoisomerase inhibitors

Topoisomerases are a group of enzymes that help the reproduction of DNA in the nucleus. Topoisomerase inhibitors damage the enzymes and stop new DNA formation.

These drugs include etoposide, used in lung cancer and testicular cancer, irinotecan (Campto), used for cancer of the large bowel, and topetecan (Hycamtin), used to treat ovarian cancer.

Combination chemotherapy

Occasionally a single cytotoxic drug will be given, but usually a combination of drugs is used. These combinations normally use several drugs that work in a variety of different ways to interfere with cell division in order to maximize the effectiveness of the treatment.

There are countless different combinations of drugs used for the numerous different types of cancer, and new regimens are being devised and tested all the time. They are often known by acronyms, based on the names of the drugs that are given. The following are examples of a few of the most widely used treatments, and the cancers for which they are given:

- CMF: cyclophosphamide, methotrexate and fluorouracil: breast cancer.

- Epi-CMF: four courses of epirubicin, given on its own, followed by four courses of CMF: breast cancer.
- FEC: fluorouracil, epirubicin and cyclophosphamide: breast cancer.
- AC: Adriamycin (the original manufacturer's name for doxorubicin) and cyclophosphamide: breast cancer.
- BEP: bleomycin, etoposide and cisplatin: testicular cancer.
- ABVD: Adriamycin, bleomycin, vinblastine and dacarbazine: a type of lymphoma called Hodgkin's disease.

Hormonal treatments

In a few types of cancer, most notably breast and prostate, hormones can play an important role in their treatment. This is because about six out of ten breast cancers, and at least nine out of ten prostate cancers, need a supply of hormone to encourage their growth. The breast cancers are dependent on the female hormone oestrogen, and the prostate cancers need the male hormone androgen. These sex hormones, which are normally present in the bloodstream, bind to a special protein in the cancer cell, called a receptor. Once the hormone has attached to the receptor, this sends signals to the nucleus of the cell, encouraging it to divide.

Simple tests can be done to see if a breast cancer contains oestrogen receptors (a tumour that does have receptors is known as ER+, one that does not is ER−; these initials being based on the American spelling of estrogen). Only an ER+ breast cancer is likely to respond to hormone treatments; ER− cancers are usually unaffected by them. Prostate cancers are not routinely tested to look for androgen receptors because they are so common that it is assumed they will always be present.

By interfering with the supply of hormone to the receptor, the growth of the cancer can often be slowed, or even reversed. This can be achieved in a number of ways, including reducing hormone production (for example, by giving drugs that suppress the ovaries, or the testicles, which make the sex hormones), or using drugs that bind to the receptors and stop the hormones from stimulating them.

Although hormonal treatments can be very important, they are not usually given at the same time as cytotoxic chemotherapy because giving the two treatments simultaneously has been shown to reduce their effectiveness.

New approaches to drug treatment of cancer

One of the limitations of cytotoxic drugs is that they cannot distinguish between cancer cells and normal cells, and this leads to unwanted side effects.

In recent years scientists have discovered that in some cancers the tumour cells contain specific proteins, or other chemicals that are unique to those cells, and that are not present in normal cells.

This means that drugs can be developed to target, and inactivate or destroy these substances. Since these proteins and chemicals are only found in cancer cells it means that the drugs have little or no effect on the normal cells.

Although this idea sounds exciting, relatively few drugs that work like this have become available so far. Most of these have been a type of compound called a monoclonal antibody. Often these have only a limited effect when used on their own, but they can sometimes improve the results of cytotoxic chemotherapy if the two types of treatment are given together.

Examples of these monoclonal antibodies include rituximab (Mabthera), which is used to treat some lymphomas; trastuzumab (Herceptin), which is used for some breast cancers; and bevacuzimab (Avastin), which is being assessed in colorectal and other cancers.

Other agents are simple chemical compounds. These include imatinib (Glivec), which is used to treat a particular type of leukaemia (chronic myeloid leukaemia); erlotinib (Tarceva), which is being assessed in some types of lung cancer; and gefitinib (Iressa), which is being looked at for lung, breast, bowel and head and neck cancer.

This is a very active and exciting area of research into cancer treatment, and the likelihood is that more drugs like these will be discovered over the next ten years.

A note about steroids

The word 'steroids' is shorthand for a family of different hormones produced by the adrenal glands (two small glands that sit on top of each of our kidneys). One group of steroids is called corticosteroids, and two synthetic versions of these hormones, called prednisolone and dexamethasone, are often used in cancer treatment.

These particular steroids can be given for a number of different reasons. Sometimes they form part of an actual chemotherapy treatment schedule. Particularly in cancers like leukaemias and lymphomas, steroids boost the effectiveness of cytotoxic drugs, and so are combined with them as part of the actual anti-cancer therapy.

Dexamethasone is also quite effective in helping to prevent or reduce the sickness caused by chemotherapy, so it is often given along with other anti-sickness drugs at the time chemotherapy is being given and for a few days afterwards.

In some types of cancer, especially brain tumours and some lung cancers, some of the symptoms are due to inflammation caused by the tumour in the tissues that surround it. Steroids help to reduce inflammation, and dexamethasone is particularly effective at doing this, so it is often given as part of the treatment for these tumours, and leads to a rapid improvement in troublesome symptoms like headache and breathlessness.

For people who have advanced, widespread cancer, steroids like prednisolone and dexamethasone can often be very effective tonics. They help increase appetite, ease sickness, improve energy levels, and make for a better quality of life with a general feeling of well-being.

Understandably, given all the publicity about various types of steroids, and their abuse by athletes and others, people often worry when their doctors tell them they will be having steroids as part of their cancer treatment. In most cases, however, the drugs are only used for a short period, a few days or weeks at a time, and when they are given in this way side effects are uncommon.

A note about bisphosphonates

The bisphosphonates are a group of drugs that help to strengthen the bones. They are increasingly being used for people who have cancers that have spread to their bones. The three conditions where they are being used most frequently are myeloma (a type of cancer that affects the marrow in the bones, and leads to bone damage), breast cancer and prostate cancer.

People often confuse these drugs with chemotherapy because they are often given as a drip into a vein in the arm once every few weeks (although they can sometimes be given as tablets). However, they are completely different from cytotoxic and other types of chemo-therapy. They also usually have very little in the way of side effects.

Bisphosphonates can be given for a number of reasons. For people who have cancers that have spread to their bones, giving these drugs can help to reduce the risk of complications like fractures and abnormally high calcium levels in the blood (hypercalcaemia). Hypercalcaemia is a quite common, and sometimes serious, compli-cation of bone secondaries. The high blood calcium levels lead to symptoms of feeling thirsty, passing a lot of urine, feeling generally ill, and sometimes becoming muddled and confused. Bisphospho-nates are good at stopping this happening (and also for treating the condition if it develops in people who have not been having the drugs).

Sometimes giving bisphosphonates can also be helpful in control-ling pain from bone secondaries. Clinical trials are also under way to see if these drugs can prevent bone secondaries developing in those women with breast cancer who are thought to be at particularly high risk of the illness spreading to their bones.

The development of bisphosphonates is a very active field in medicine, and new drugs are being introduced all the time; some of the most widely used are pamidronate (Aredia), clodronate (Bone-fos), etidronate (Didronel), zoledronic acid (Zometa) and ibandronic acid (Bondronat).

Incidentally, bisphosphonates are also used in a number of non-cancerous bone conditions, like some types of osteoporosis (bone thinning), so the fact that someone is on one of these drugs does not necessarily mean that they have got cancer.

Costs and 'postcode prescribing' in chemotherapy

Chemotherapy can be very expensive. Some of the older drugs, which have been available for the last 30 or 40 years, cost only a few pounds, but some of the newer drugs cost hundreds of pounds – and sometimes more than £1,000 for a single dose. Fortunately, these costs are often covered by the NHS, and the treatment is free of charge for anyone who needs it.

But the high cost of some of the newer drugs has led to worries about 'postcode prescribing'. This means that a particular drug may be available in some hospitals, but not in others, simply because of what can be afforded in different parts of the country. Therefore the treatment you are offered may depend on where you live.

This was a real problem a few years ago, but in 1999 the National Institute for Clinical Excellence (NICE) was set up. Part of NICE's work is to look at all new drugs, including cancer treatments, and to decide whether they are likely to offer a worthwhile improvement in treatment. If NICE feels that the drug is going to be helpful, and approves it, then it has to be provided for anyone who needs it. This means that nowadays, wherever you live in the UK, you should be able to get the best possible drug treatment for your cancer, regardless of cost.

4
What is involved?

The chemotherapy that someone might need varies enormously, depending on the type of cancer they have, and the stage of the disease (whether it is early, or more advanced and widespread). At its simplest, treatment involves no more than taking a tablet once a day; at its most complex, it may mean many months of intensive treatment as an in-patient on a hospital ward. However, these are extremes, and for most people treatment will mean a number of visits as an out-patient or day-patient to a Chemotherapy Unit over a period of about six months.

These Chemotherapy Units are run by specially trained staff and are only available at certain hospitals. This may mean that your local hospital will not be able to do the treatment and you may have to travel some distance to get to your nearest Chemotherapy Unit.

Who gives the treatment?

Cancer chemotherapy is a very specialized area of medicine, so although your initial care may have been under a surgeon or physician, they will usually refer you to another of their consultant colleagues if you need cytotoxic treatment. Most chemotherapy is given either by a clinical oncologist (a consultant who is qualified to give both chemotherapy and radiotherapy), or a medical oncologist (who specializes exclusively in drug treatment of cancer). If you have a leukaemia or lymphoma, your chemotherapy might be given by a consultant called a clinical haematologist.

Although the consultant will decide what treatment you need, and be responsible for your overall care while you are receiving that treatment, your chemotherapy will usually be given by specialist chemotherapy nurses, and they will look after many of your day-to-day needs, and any problems you may have, throughout the treatment.

Starting off

When you first meet the specialist who will look after you during your chemotherapy, he or she will usually start by going through your medical history and the details of your present problem. They will probably also want to do a physical examination, and check on the results of any tests – such as scans or x-rays – that you may have had.

Your doctor will then discuss your treatment with you. He or she may make a clear-cut recommendation, based on what they think is best for you, or it may be that there are different options for treatment, and that when these have been explained you can actually choose which ones you would prefer.

Usually, if there is a choice involved, you would be given time to make a decision, and wouldn't be expected to make up your mind there and then.

In outlining your treatment the doctor should explain why you need it, and what is involved, including how the treatment will be given (tablets, or injections, or drips), whether it will mean a stay in hospital at any time, how often it needs to be done, how long it will go on for, and what side effects you might experience.

This first visit is obviously very important and it is a very good idea to have someone with you, a friend or relative, who can help you remember what was said, and compare notes with you afterwards; even though you will usually be given some written information at the time, it still helps to have someone who you can talk things through with at home. Another thing that is worthwhile is to make a list of questions you want to ask about your cancer and its treatment before you see your specialist. The likelihood is that he or she will answer most of your queries while explaining matters to you, but you can use your list to check on this and to prompt you about any unanswered questions. Having things written down is a wise precaution because, however carefully you prepare, your mind can often go blank during a consultation.

Once you have agreed on the proposed treatment with your specialist you will usually be asked to sign a consent form. This confirms that you feel everything has been properly explained to you and that you are willing to go ahead with the chemotherapy.

The doctor will then arrange the date for your first treatment, but you may need some routine blood tests, or other tests, before this can be confirmed. Depending on the drugs you are going to be given, these tests may be done to check various things, including your blood count, kidney function and liver function, and to make sure that your heart is working well (with an electrocardiogram (ECG) test). The doctor will probably also measure your height and weight, as these are used to work out the actual doses of the drugs that you will be given.

The chemotherapy nurses

Before you actually start your chemotherapy you may well have a visit arranged for you to look round the Chemotherapy Unit, and to meet the specialist nurses who will be looking after you during your treatment.

This preliminary visit can be useful in a number of ways: it obviously gives you the chance to see where you will have your treatment, and get a feel for what is likely to be involved, and to meet the people who will be doing this for you. But it also gives you the chance to ask any questions you have thought of since you saw your specialist.

At this preliminary visit you may well be given some more written information about your treatment. These days, this often includes your own 'handheld record'. This is a booklet that includes details about the Chemotherapy Unit, including contact telephone numbers in case you have any problems in between your visits. It usually also has a diary section where you can record your own details of the treatment, your blood test results and any other notes.

Having chemotherapy

As I said earlier, very occasionally chemotherapy involves no more than taking tablets on a regular basis, but this is uncommon and most treatments involve having drugs given directly into a vein. This may mean having injections over a matter of a few minutes, or having an infusion (a drip) over an hour or so, or a continuous infusion, where the drug is given through a pump over days, or weeks. Nowadays, if you are going to have a lot of injections and blood tests you may be offered a venous line (explained below) to make this easier for you.

Chemotherapy treatment is usually given on an out-patient basis. The pattern of your visits will vary with different types of chemo- therapy – the drugs might be given once every three or four weeks,

27

or given over a few days in succession, followed by a gap of a week or two before the next course. Overall treatment may continue anywhere from a few weeks to a year or more, although most treatments last about five or six months.

Before each treatment you will normally have a blood test. This checks your blood count, looking at your haemoglobin level (checking whether you are anaemic or not), the number of white blood cells (which prevent you getting infections), and the number of platelets (if these drop too low, you are at risk of getting abnormal bleeding). All these can be affected by chemotherapy, so it is important to make sure that their levels are safe before the drugs are given.

With some treatments you will need to take some tablets or medicines a few hours before each chemotherapy session, as a 'pre-med', to prevent or reduce side effects. You will usually also have drugs given, either into the vein or as tablets, at the time your chemotherapy is given, to help to prevent any unpleasant after-effects. There is also likely to be a supply of tablets for you to take home, to have in the next few days after treatment, in order to stop any nausea or vomiting. With some drugs there may be other medicines as well, to stop other side effects occurring.

Venous lines

Having a course of chemotherapy usually involves a lot of needles, both for all the blood tests that need to be done and for giving the drugs themselves.

Having a venous line offers an alternative to this. The line is a fine hollow silicone rubber tube, or catheter, which is inserted into a vein and stays in place throughout the time of your course of chemotherapy. Two types of line are used: a central line or a PICC line.

The central line is inserted through the skin just below your collar bone, into a large vein called the subclavian vein, and threaded along this until its tip lies in another large vein, the superior vena cava, just above your heart. Central lines are also sometimes known by the names of the manufacturers of the lines, the two main ones being Hickman and Groshong.

A PICC line (also known as a peripheral line) is inserted through one of the large veins near the bend of your elbow, and threaded along this, through the subclavian vein and into the superior vena cava. Once in place, the line can be used for taking blood for any tests you need during your treatment and for giving all the drugs that would normally have to be injected into a vein, or given through a drip. The line is usually quite comfortable and can stay in place for a year or more if necessary.

Putting in the line is quite a simple procedure. Placing a PICC line can be done as an out-patient and does not need a general anaesthetic. The skin where the line is to be inserted is numbed with some local anaesthetic, and threading the line through the veins is usually quite painless, so you shouldn't have much discomfort when this is being done. The insertion only takes a few minutes and you have a chest x-ray immediately afterwards to make sure that the tip of the line is in the right place. Putting a central line in is very similar, but sometimes this may be done with a short general anaesthetic rather than a local anaesthetic.

Once the line is in place it is important that it doesn't get blocked. To prevent this it will have to be flushed through with special fluid once or twice a week. Your nurses may ask you to come up to the hospital to have this done, or they may arrange for a nurse to visit you at home. Sometimes it may be possible for them to teach you, or a friend or relative, how to flush the line.

Normally lines are very trouble-free. The most common problems that do occur are infections, and blockages from small blood clots. Your chemotherapy nurses will always know what to do if you have any difficulties with your line.

Venous lines can be very helpful for people who are going to need a lot of injections, blood tests and drips during their treatment; they are also valuable for people who can't bear the thought of needles, and for people who have 'poor' veins which are difficult to extract blood from, or for injecting fluids. Lines are also essential for people who are having their chemotherapy continuously, through a pump, over a period of days or weeks.

When it comes to removing the line, this is very simple. It is done in the out-patient clinic, with just a local anaesthetic to avoid any discomfort, and only takes a few minutes.

Although the idea of having a line that stays in place for some months may seem a little strange, once it is in place it is usually trouble-free. People soon get used to them and find that they don't really interfere with their everyday lives.

Implantable ports

Implantable ports are a variation on venous lines. The line is placed in a similar way, but instead of the end of it coming out on the skin, it ends in a subcutaneous port. This is a small soft plastic bubble, between about 2.5 and 4 centimetres (1 to $1\frac{1}{2}$ inches) across, which lies just under the surface of the skin. This means it is less obvious than a central or PICC line, and appears as just a little bump under the skin. It is usually placed near the top of the front of the chest.

Like central lines, implantable ports may be inserted either when you are an out-patient, with a local anaesthetic, or occasionally as a day-patient, if a general anaesthetic is used. They also need regular flushing to stop them becoming blocked.

Implantable ports (which are also known as portocaths) can be used just like the venous lines: for taking blood tests, or giving chemotherapy or blood transfusions or other intravenous fluids.

Infusion pumps

When a chemotherapy drug is given into a vein it is usual to set up a drip, with a bag of fluid, on a drip stand, which trickles through a tube into the vein. The drug may either be given as an injection into the tubing of the drip, or it may be mixed with the fluid in the bag and run in as an infusion.

Depending on the treatment that is being given, the drip may last for anywhere from a few minutes to a few hours. But some chemotherapy treatments require the drugs to be given into a vein over a matter of days or even weeks. For these long infusions, a portable pump can be used, along with a venous line. The pump is a battery-driven device that holds a syringe, containing the chemotherapy drug. This is attached to the end of the venous line, and very slowly the pump squeezes a trickle of the drug into the vein. Once the infusion is complete, then the pump is very simply disconnected.

Pumps vary in size, but are usually little bigger than a mobile phone. They can be worn in a special 'holster', meaning that they are easy to carry around, and not very obvious. This means that treatment can continue when you are at home, and there should be very little effect on your normal day-to-day activities while the infusion is in progress.

Lumbar puncture

Very occasionally, most often with certain types of leukaemia, it may be necessary to give chemotherapy drugs into the space around the spinal cord, the major nerve that runs through the bones of the back (the vertebrae). This is so that the drug can reach parts of the nervous system that it might not get to if it was given by an ordinary infusion into a vein. This type of treatment is called epidural chemotherapy.

This involves having a lumbar puncture. This can be done as an out-patient, or a day-patient. It involves having an injection of local anaesthetic into the skin over the lower part of your spine. Once the area is numb, a needle is then slipped in between the vertebrae, into the spinal canal. When the needle is in place, the drug is injected over a period of a few minutes. The needle is then removed. Usually you will be asked to lie still, on your back, for an hour or so after the procedure, before you go home. You may have a mild headache for up to 24 hours after a lumbar puncture.

5

What are the side effects?

In this chapter we will look at some of the main side effects of chemotherapy, and in the next chapter we will talk about how these can be prevented or reduced.

When someone first hears they need chemotherapy, their biggest worry is usually the side effects of the treatment. Chemotherapy has a reputation for causing severe distress and disruption. While this can occasionally be true, it is important to make a few general points about the impact of chemotherapy, before going into a bit more detail about side effects.

Chemotherapy is not a single type of treatment. What is actually involved in having chemotherapy varies enormously depending on the type of cancer you have, and the stage that the cancer has reached. As mentioned earlier, at one extreme, chemotherapy may be no more than taking a tablet once a day, with virtually no side effects at all; at the other end of the spectrum, it may involve a year or more of intensive treatment, with long stays in hospital and possibly severe, even dangerous, complications. For most people, however, treatment will mean a number of visits to the Chemotherapy Unit, as an out-patient or a day-patient, over four to six months, with the possibility of some temporarily troublesome, but not very upsetting, side effects.

Another thing is that people react differently to the same treatment. Two people can be having an identical type of chemotherapy, for exactly the same type of cancer, and be of similar age, with a similar level of general fitness, and whereas one will sail through treatment with virtually no problems, the other may experience a number of side effects, and their treatment may be quite a struggle.

This means that hearing how other people have coped with their chemotherapy isn't necessarily a good guide to what will happen to you. First, they will probably have had a completely different type of treatment, and second, even if they have had similar drugs to you, their experience of the treatment may well be completely different to your own.

Certainly, before you start your treatment, your oncologist, and the nurses who will be giving you chemotherapy, should have explained to you all the common side effects that might occur with that treatment, and also have given you an idea of how likely it is that you will experience those side effects, and how troublesome they might be. They should also reassure you that they will give you help and support to deal with any problems that do occur. So, although no one will be able to predict in advance exactly how you will react to the treatment, you will have some idea of the sort of things that could happen, and know that there will be sympathetic nurses and doctors, with expert knowledge, who will help you to cope if you do run into difficulties.

Common side effects of treatment

There are many different chemotherapy drugs, and many different combinations of these drugs are used in cancer treatment. This means that the likely side effects vary considerably depending on the drugs that are needed, and the doses that are used. Having said this, there are some side effects that occur much more often than others. These include changes to your blood count (bone marrow suppression), sickness (nausea and vomiting), tiredness, hair loss (alopecia), mouth soreness and dryness, and reduced fertility.

Changes to the blood count

Our blood contains three essential types of cell:

- The red blood cells (red corpuscles): these carry oxygen to the tissues.
- The white blood cells (white corpuscles): these help to protect us against infections.
- The platelets: these prevent bleeding.

All these cells are made by stem cells in the bone marrow, the spongy material that is inside many of the bones in our bodies. These stem cells are very sensitive to the drugs used in chemotherapy, and will often be damaged by a dose of chemotherapy, which leads to fewer blood cells being produced.

If your stem cells are making fewer red blood cells than normal, this causes anaemia, making you feel tired, and sometimes causes other symptoms, such as breathlessness. If too few white cells are being made, you usually don't feel any different, but it does mean your resistance is low, and you are more likely to pick up infections.

If too few platelets are produced, then you are more at risk of bruising easily, and getting abnormal bleeding.

Normally the effect of a dose of chemotherapy on the bone marrow cells is temporary. The changes come on a few days after treatment, reaching a peak at about ten to fourteen days, and then recovering over the next week or so.

A simple blood test, the full blood count, gives a quick and accurate measurement of all the different cells in the blood.

The production of white blood cells is the most sensitive to chemotherapy. If a blood count is done one or two weeks after a dose of chemotherapy, it will usually show a fall in the number of white blood cells. Changes to the red cells, and platelets, generally occur more slowly, and are only likely to show up after several courses of chemotherapy (and very often are not affected at all, throughout the entire treatment).

When you are having chemotherapy you will have a full blood count before you start treatment, to make sure your bone marrow is working properly, and that all your blood cells are at a normal level. The blood count will then be repeated before each new course, or dose, of chemotherapy, during treatment, to make sure that your cell counts have recovered, and are at a safe level, before the next treatment is given.

If the blood count has not recovered sufficiently, the next treatment may be delayed, or the dose of the drugs may be reduced so that they do not damage the bone marrow cells any further.

Nausea and vomiting

Many chemotherapy treatments can make people feel sick. Very often this is bad enough to actually make them vomit. The nausea comes on a few hours after having the drugs. It is usually at its worst during the first two days after the chemotherapy has been given, and then settles quite quickly over another day or two.

The chances of experiencing sickness, and its severity, varies enormously with different chemotherapy drugs. Some cause virtually no upset, whereas others can lead to very unpleasant sickness.

Happily, over the last ten years or so, the prevention and treatment of nausea and vomiting caused by chemotherapy has improved quite dramatically. This has been as a result of the introduction of new anti-sickness drugs, which have proved far more effective than older treatments.

It is important to realize that this change has taken place. Many people still remember friends or relatives who had their chemotherapy in the 1970s or 1980s and suffered very badly from sickness and vomiting, but these days this sort of problem is really very uncommon. You may feel a little bit queasy, and a bit off your food for a day or so after each treatment, but this is usually the worst that you are likely to experience.

Tiredness or fatigue

For many people, tiredness is the main problem they experience as a result of their cancer. This tiredness can have many causes; just having a cancer can often make you feel very weary. But there is no doubt that chemotherapy can also lead to tiredness.

The tiredness, or fatigue, due to chemotherapy usually comes on during the first week or two of treatment, and often gradually gets more apparent as the course of treatment continues. Once the chemotherapy is over, the sense of fatigue slowly reduces, but it can take anywhere from a month or two to more than a year before it completely disappears.

The tiredness is more likely if you are having, or have recently had, other treatments, like surgery or radiotherapy.

The feeling of fatigue can be very difficult to cope with. It can make even the slightest effort seem like a major task. Not only is there often a complete lack of energy, but the tiredness can also interfere with other things – like your memory, your sleeping pattern and your sex life. It may also lead to symptoms like breathlessness and loss of appetite. It can be difficult to feel interested in anything, and you often feel quite low and depressed.

Because it is not something that is easily measurable – like a change in your blood count – or not very obvious – like sickness and vomiting – fatigue has in the past tended to be overlooked as a side effect of treatment. But nowadays doctors and nurses are aware that it can be a big problem for many people, and there is often a lot that can be done to help. So, if your treatment does make you feel very tired, do let your medical and nursing team know this.

Hair loss

For many people, the idea of having chemotherapy means that you must lose your hair. In fact, the risk of hair loss is linked directly to which drugs you are given. With some chemotherapy drugs, hair loss almost always happens, whereas with others it is virtually unknown.

Your doctors and nurses should be able to let you know how likely alopecia (hair loss) is with your particular treatment, and what can be done to reduce the risk, or cope with the problem when it develops.

When hair loss occurs, it usually develops about three to four weeks after starting treatment. Sometimes, once it starts, it can progress very rapidly, with almost complete hair loss within a day or two; with other types of treatment, it may be more a case of gradual thinning of the hair over several months.

Scalp hair is the most sensitive to the effects of chemotherapy, because it grows more rapidly than hair on other parts of the body. But sometimes the drugs will cause loss of eyebrows, eyelashes, under-arm hair, and pubic hair as well.

It is important to remember that, however much hair you lose during your treatment, it will grow back again afterwards (indeed, sometimes it even starts to grow while you are still having the drugs). Normally the hair begins to reappear a month or so after the end of chemotherapy, and is back completely within three to six months. Often, however, it comes back with a different colour and appearance – a grey/black, 'pepper and salt' colouring, with a quite thick texture, and a slightly curly or wavy look is very common.

Sore mouth

Having a sore mouth during chemotherapy is quite common. When this happens, it usually comes on a few days after the drugs have been given and settles within about a week.

If it does happen, the soreness can vary considerably in its severity. Often it is no more than a slight discomfort, but sometimes it can be very uncomfortable, and mouth ulcers can develop. Because your white blood cell count may be low at this time, the soreness may be aggravated by the development of fungal infections in the mouth, a condition known as oral thrush, or *oral monilia*. This leads to whitish patches on the tongue and the lining of the mouth.

When mouth soreness develops it can also affect your sense of taste, so that things taste different, or you may find you cannot taste things so well.

Reduced fertility

As with other side effects, the risk of any effect on fertility is related to which drugs are used, and the doses given, and the length of time the treatment goes on for. Some chemotherapy treatments carry a very high risk of infertility, whereas with others there is almost no risk.

For women, the likelihood of becoming infertile also relates to their age. The chemotherapy drugs that cause infertility do so by stopping the ovaries from making the female hormones that regulate the menstrual cycle. This leads to an early menopause, with the periods stopping, and often the onset of symptoms like hot flushes, vaginal dryness and mood changes that are associated with the change of life. The risk of loss of ovarian activity with chemotherapy increases the closer a woman is to the natural menopause, so for a woman in her early twenties the chances of infertility with a particular type of treatment will be less than for a woman in her mid-forties.

Sometimes chemotherapy leads to a temporary loss of ovarian activity, so the periods stop during treatment, and for anywhere from three to eighteen months afterwards, but then can start again.

For men, the risk relates almost entirely to which drugs are used. But in some types of cancer, in particular cancer of the testicle, a reduced level of fertility, with a lower than normal sperm count, may actually be part of their condition even before they begin any treatment.

Because of the unpredictability of the effects of some types of chemotherapy on fertility, it would be wrong to think that having treatment acts as a reliable form of contraception. If you are practising birth control, then you should certainly continue this while you are having your chemotherapy.

More specific side effects

There are a number of side effects of chemotherapy which, although important, and occasionally serious, are limited to just a handful of the more commonly used cytotoxic drugs. These side effects include nerve damage, damage to the heart and lungs, kidney damage, allergic reactions and skin and eye complications.

Nerve damage

When this happens it usually takes the form of a peripheral neuropathy. This affects the nerves in the arms and legs, usually beginning in the hands and feet. The first symptom is tingling, or pins and needles, in the fingers or toes. This gradually spreads to the rest of the hands and feet, and, if nothing is done, will go on to affect the rest of the limbs. As the condition progresses, numbness of the affected areas will develop, and this leads to some loss of co-ordination, making fine movements like undoing buttons, or tying shoelaces, more difficult. In its more advanced stages there may be weakness of the muscles in the arms and legs.

Peripheral neuropathy is a recognized complication of treatment with three groups of chemotherapy drugs: the Vinca alkaloids (which include vincristine, vinblastine, vindesine and vinorelbine), the platinum compounds (cisplatin, carboplatin, and oxaliplatin), and the taxanes (paclitaxel and docetaxel).

Another type of nerve damage that is limited to the platinum drugs, especially cisplatin, leads to problems with hearing. This begins as noises in the ear, whistling, buzzing or ringing sounds (which doctors call 'tinnitus'). This can lead on to an actual loss of hearing and deafness.

Both peripheral neuropathy and hearing problems (ototoxicity) only come on very gradually, over weeks or months, and are related to the doses of the drugs that are being given. Doctors are very well aware of these side effects, and will regularly ask if you are noticing any numbness, pins and needles, or have any ringing or buzzing in your ears if you are being given these compounds. If you do notice any of these symptoms, do let your medical team know, and then they will be able to adjust your treatment before any harm is done.

Damage to the heart

A group of drugs called anthracyclines, which include doxorubicin and epirubicin, can cause damage to the heart muscle. This can lead to weakness of the heart muscle, and heart failure. This only occurs after quite large amounts of the drug have been given over many months, and these days most of the dose schedules using these drugs ensure that the total amount of the drug given throughout the course of treatment is well within the safe level, where heart damage is extremely unlikely. It is usual, however, for people who are going to be given one of these drugs to have a routine heart test and ECG, just to make sure that their heart is quite healthy before they start treatment.

The group of drugs called taxanes (paclitaxel and docetaxel) can also affect the heart. They can interfere with the control of heart rhythm leading to an irregular heart beat. Usually, even if this happens, it does not cause any real symptoms or problems. The taxanes, especially docetaxel, can also lead to fluid retention, which shows itself by causing swelling of the ankles and lower legs (ankle oedema). Although ankle oedema is one sign of heart failure, the fluid retention caused by taxanes does not seem to be directly related to any effect on the heart.

Lung damage

This is very uncommon, but two drugs – bleomycin and busulphan – when given at high doses, can lead to thickening of the tissues in the lung (lung fibrosis), which can lead to shortness of breath. Since it has been realized that this can happen, the doses of the drugs given these days are usually well below the levels where this complication might develop.

Kidney damage

The platinum compounds, in particular cisplatin, can damage the kidneys, leading to partial kidney failure. Because of this, it is normal before someone has treatment with a platinum drug to do tests to check how well their kidneys are working. When this has been done, the drug can be prescribed at a safe level to ensure that the risk of any injury to the kidneys is minimal. Usually simple blood tests, and sometimes more complex tests of renal (kidney) function, will be done during the course of treatment, before each dose of the drug, to make sure there is no evidence of kidney damage developing.

With some other drugs, where removal of the chemical from the body by the kidneys is very important, tests of renal function may be done before treatment starts, to ensure that the kidneys can handle the drug, even though the drug itself does not cause any damage to the kidney.

Allergic reactions

Some drugs, including the taxanes (paclitaxel and docetaxel) and bleomycin, may cause allergic or hypersensitivity reactions. These show up as fevers, or shivers and shakes, often with a feeling of weakness or sickness, which come on within a few minutes to an hour or so after starting the drug. Usually this problem can be avoided by giving other drugs before the chemotherapy, which will prevent an allergic reaction occurring.

Skin damage

Most chemotherapy drugs are given through a drip into a vein. Even when the drug is given very carefully, by trained skilled nurses, small amounts of the drug may occasionally leak outside the vein, into the surrounding soft tissues. This is called extravasation. With most drugs, extravasation is not a problem, and will only cause some very slight brief discomfort at most. With a few drugs, however, any leakage into the tissues around the vein can cause quite severe inflammation, with redness, swelling and soreness. This comes on almost immediately after the extravasation has occurred, and, depending on the drug and the amount that has leaked into the tissues, may take days, or even weeks, to settle down.

The drugs most likely to cause irritation and skin damage when they leak are anthracyclines (doxorubicin and epirubicin) and the Vinca alkaloids (vincristine, vinblastine, vindesine and vinorelbine).

The risk of this kind of damage can be avoided by having a central line or PICC line for your drug administration, but even if you are having your drugs through an ordinary drip into a vein in your arm, then it is still a very uncommon problem. If it does occur, then putting ice packs on the area and having injections of steroids under the skin where the leakage has occurred will reduce the immediate discomfort, and lessen the risk of any lasting skin damage or scarring. Using an anti-inflammatory cream on the affected area for a week or so afterwards can also help.

A completely different type of skin damage can occur with the drugs fluorouracil and capecitabine. These can lead to a condition known as hand-foot syndrome. In hand–foot syndrome the skin on the palms of the hands and soles of the feet becomes red and sore, and may actually begin to blister and peel. It usually only comes on gradually, with higher doses of the drugs, and adjusting the dose will usually ease the problem. Sometimes taking tablets of Vitamin B6 (called pyridoxine) can help, and your doctor may prescribe these for you.

Eye complications

Serious eye problems are very rare indeed with chemotherapy drugs, but some drugs, in particular fluorouracil, can lead to a feeling of soreness or grittiness in the eyes, with watering of the eyes as well. Soothing eye drops will usually ease this symptom.

Diarrhoea and constipation

A few drugs, in particular irinotecan and cisplatin, may cause diarrhoea, and occasionally this can be severe. If this is likely to happen, your doctors and nurses will usually warn you about it, and give you a supply of tablets or capsules that you can take if the problem develops. They will also advise you that drinking plenty of fluids, to make sure you don't get dehydrated, is important if you do get diarrhoea.

Constipation may occur if you are having Vinca alkaloid drugs (vincristine, vinblastine, vinorelbine or vindesine). It is also a side effect of some of the drugs used to prevent sickness, so you may find you are a bit constipated in the first day or two after having your chemotherapy. Once again, drinking plenty of fluids helps to reduce the likelihood of a problem, and eating plenty of fresh fruit and fibre is a good idea.

Cancer formation

Over the 60 years that chemotherapy has been used, there have been occasional reports suggesting that giving cytotoxic drugs can actually lead to a risk of developing another cancer later in life. The likelihood of chemotherapy leading to cancer formation has been the subject of a very great deal of research. This has shown that although it is impossible to say there is absolutely no risk, if there *is* a chance of cytotoxic chemotherapy drugs leading to cancer development, it is a very, very small risk indeed, and these minute risks have been far outweighed by the benefits of treatment.

6

Coping with the side effects

The last chapter has described a number of the side effects that can occur with chemotherapy. Happily, for many people, there will be relatively few problems during their treatment. However, for others there may be troublesome and unpleasant symptoms, and this chapter describes how the risk of the most common side effects can be reduced, and, when they do occur, how to cope with them to keep any upset to a minimum.

Infection

Nearly all chemotherapy drugs have an effect on the bone marrow, which leads to a reduction in the number of white cells circulating in the blood. As the white blood cells are the body's main line of defence against infections, this means that you may be more at risk of picking up an infection while you are having chemotherapy.

How badly the bone marrow is affected depends on the drugs that you are given and the doses that are used. Typically, the white cell count in the blood begins to fall about five to seven days after a dose of cytotoxics, and will reach its lowest level about two weeks after the treatment. After that, the count recovers and will be more or less back to normal by the end of the third week. You will always have a blood test before the next dose of drugs is given in order to ensure that your blood count has recovered sufficiently for it to be safe to carry on with the treatment.

Your doctors and nurses should warn you about the risk of infection while you are on treatment, and explain how high that risk is in your particular case. The usual advice would be that if, at any time during treatment, you get a temperature of more than 38°C (100.5°F), or if you develop symptoms suggesting an infection – like shivering, a sore throat, or a cough and shortness of breath, or cystitis (stinging and burning when you pass urine and wanting to pass water more often than usual), or if you simply suddenly feel unwell – then you should let your hospital know immediately. There will always be someone available to see you and advise what to do. Usually they will talk to you, and probably examine you, and take a blood test. The hospital team should always give you contact phone numbers so that you can get in touch at any time, night or day, and at weekends, if you are worried – do make sure you have these, and know where they are should you need them.

If you do develop an infection, then this can normally be treated as an out-patient with a course of antibiotics. But sometimes, for more severe infections, or if your blood count is very low, you may need to go into hospital for a few days for intensive antibiotic therapy, with the drugs being given through a drip into a vein. You may also have injections of growth factors (G-CSF, or granulocyte colony stimulating factors); these are compounds that stimulate the bone marrow to produce more white blood cells and help speed the recovery of the blood count. They are usually given as very small injections under the skin once or twice a day.

Occasionally your time in hospital may involve something called reverse barrier nursing, where you are in a room on your own and when people come in they will have to wear gowns and masks, and either put on gloves or use special antibacterial hand washes. All this is done to protect you from picking up any further infections, and is usually only necessary for a day or two until your white blood cell count begins to recover.

If you have had an infection after a dose of chemotherapy, then your doctors may give you antibiotics to take before and during your remaining courses of the drugs to prevent any further episodes. Less commonly, they may use injections of growth factors, G-CSF, during your remaining courses of treatment to try and boost your white blood cell levels.

Sometimes, if your medical team think that the drugs you are going to be given will put you at high risk of picking up an infection, then they may start you on antibiotics before you begin your chemotherapy, to try to stop this happening.

There are a number of things that you can do to help reduce your chances of getting an infection while you are having chemotherapy. These include:

- Avoid friends or family members who have an obvious infection, like a bad cold or flu, or children with illnesses such as measles, mumps or chickenpox. Chickenpox is particularly important as the virus that causes this is the same one that causes shingles (herpes zoster), and people who are having chemotherapy are particularly likely to get shingles.

- Avoid very crowded places where you will have to spend time close to large numbers of people, because you can never tell if any of them might be carrying an infection you could catch.
- Avoid swimming or other sports where you have to share changing rooms and showers with other people.
- Be very particular about your personal hygiene. Bath or shower at least once a day, always wash your hands thoroughly after going to the toilet, and before preparing any food or cooking. Try to make sure you have your own flannel, towels and soaps, and don't share with other members of the family.
- Take care with oral hygiene too, because mouth infections are common while you are having chemotherapy. Drink plenty of fluids (at least 2 litres (4 pints) a day) as this will keep your mouth moist and reduce the risk of an infection. Brush your teeth at least twice a day, with a soft brush. Take advice from your doctors and nurses as to whether using a mouthwash as well might be a good idea.
- Drink plenty of fluids as this helps to reduce the chances of getting cystitis. There is also some evidence that having a glass of cranberry juice each morning and evening can help to stop you picking up a urine infection.
- If your doctors and nurses think you have a very high risk of getting an infection, or if your white blood count goes very low, they may give you advice about what you should, or rather should not, be eating. This usually means avoiding raw foods, like salads, or foods that might naturally contain bacteria, like cheeses and yoghurts. Takeaway foods are also not a good idea.

One thing people often ask about is whether they should have a flu jab. Having a flu jab won't do any harm, but if your white cell count is very low, and your immunity is reduced, it may not be very effective, and may not give you very much protection against getting influenza. The best thing, if you are going to have the jab, is to have it about two weeks before you first start the treatment. If you decide to have it after you have started chemotherapy, then try to get it at a time when your white blood count is as near normal as possible (just before a course of treatment is due). Your nurses will be able to advise you of the best time, and could arrange a blood test so that you can be sure the white cell level is reasonable.

Sickness: nausea and vomiting

Along with hair loss, sickness is the thing that most people fear about chemotherapy. Until the early 1990s, this was a major problem and could often be very difficult to control, but the introduction of a new group of anti-sickness drugs (anti-emetics) called the 5HT3 antagonists brought about a huge improvement, so that nowadays severe sickness is something that only a very small minority of people experience.

The likelihood and severity of sickness depends on the drugs that are being given. Some cytotoxic drugs are much more likely to cause sickness than others. There is also evidence that some people are more vulnerable to chemotherapy-induced nausea and vomiting: women are more at risk than men; younger people are more at risk than older people; and a history of motion sickness means you are more likely to have problems.

The best way to manage chemotherapy-induced sickness is to prevent it happening in the first place. This means that with any treatment where nausea and vomiting are anticipated, you will be given anti-emetics routinely before the cytotoxic drugs. As most chemotherapy drugs are given through a drip into a vein, this usually involves having the anti-emetics injected into the drip immediately before the cytotoxics. You will then usually have a supply of anti-emetic tablets to take for a day or two afterwards.

The effectiveness of anti-emetics can be increased by giving a steroid drug called dexamethasone at the same time. People sometimes worry about 'having steroids' because of the risk of side effects, but as the drug is only given for a few doses during each course of treatment, the risk of any problems is very small indeed. One thing to mention is that dexamethasone has a tendency to keep you awake, so do try to take the last dose of the day before about 5 p.m., or you could have trouble getting off to sleep.

Although the worst of any sickness from chemotherapy passes within a day or two, feelings of queasiness, and sometimes actually being sick, can persist for a week or even longer. These troublesome, but less severe, symptoms can often be controlled by milder anti-emetics, which once again can be taken as tablets for up to a fortnight after treatment.

So a typical pattern for anti-emetic administration would be to have a dose of a 5HT3 antagonist, like ondansetron (Zofran) or granisetron (Kytril), along with a dose of dexamethasone given into a vein just before the chemotherapy is given. These would be followed by tablets of the 5HT3 antagonist and steroid to take regularly twice a day for the next two or three days. There would then be a supply of another type of anti-emetic, typically metoclopramide (Maxolon) or domperidone (Motilium), to take as and when necessary to relieve any feelings of sickness over the next week or so. This schedule will stop sickness altogether, or keep it to a very low, and tolerable, level for the great majority of people. But everyone is different, and sometimes these measures will not be enough. If this is the case, then your doctors and nurses will be able to adjust the doses or timing of your anti-sickness drugs, or add in other anti-emetics to try to give you the maximum possible relief.

Although 5HT3 antagonists are very effective at preventing and relieving sickness, some people do find they get side effects from them. The most common of these are constipation and headache. These can usually be relieved very easily, with a simple laxative like Senokot, or a simple painkiller like paracetamol. If you do think you are getting side effects, then mention it to your chemotherapy nurses who will be able to advise you how to ease them.

A recent development is the introduction of a drug called aprepitant (Emend). This works in a different way to other anti-sickness drugs and seems especially good at preventing the delayed sickness that comes on a day or two after treatment, which is a particular feature of some drugs, especially one called cisplatin. It is given as a tablet, along with a 5HT3 antagonist and dexamethasone.

As well as taking the anti-emetic medication you have been given by your chemotherapy team, there are a number of things you can try for yourself if you are feeling sick. These include the following suggestions:

- Avoid greasy, fatty or very spicy foods.
- Take ginger, since this helps to ease sickness; try nibbling a ginger biscuit or drinking ginger ale or ginger beer.
- Avoid big meals, and eat little and often with light bites and snacks.
- If you feel sick first thing in the morning, keep a couple of dry biscuits by your bed and try to eat one before you get up.
- Make sure you have plenty of fresh air; keep a window open if you can, especially when cooking.

- If cooking smells upset you, try to get someone else to prepare your meals, or opt for cold food, with salads and sandwiches.
- Some people find that sea-bands can be helpful. These are bands that you strap on round your wrists. They are fitted with a button that gently presses on the skin over an acupressure point on the inner surface of the wrist. You can buy these sea-bands at any chemist.

Tiredness or fatigue

Profound tiredness, or fatigue, is a very common problem during chemotherapy. It is thought that four out of five people will experience fatigue on some days during their treatment, and for about one in three it will be present most of the time. Although it is something that affects the majority of people, doctors have been slow to realize how important this tiredness is, and have concentrated on more obvious side effects like sickness and the risk of infection. This means there has been relatively little research into the causes and treatment of chemotherapy-related fatigue.

All of us get tired from time to time, but the fatigue that comes with chemotherapy can be much more severe than this: you may feel tired even when you are resting. Everyday activities – like washing yourself or making a cup of tea – can seem like major tasks; concentrating on things is difficult; and meeting other people – even close friends and family – can be an ordeal.

An important thing to remember is that this tiredness is a very common feature of chemotherapy and it does not mean that the cancer is coming back, or getting worse, nor does it mean that things are going wrong with your treatment.

Although chemotherapy itself does cause weariness, there can be other factors that might make the feeling worse. These include:

- Anaemia: this is a common complication of cancer, and its treatment.
- The presence of an infection.
- Being clinically depressed.
- Being in pain.

All these are things that can often readily be corrected. So if you are feeling very tired, do mention it to your doctor and nurses so that they can check for these problems and arrange any treatment that may be necessary.

Many people don't tell their medical team when they feel worn out and lethargic, because they think that this is only to be expected, and don't want to be a bother – but if you don't let them know, then they won't be able to help you, so do speak up.

Anaemia can usually be rapidly reversed by a simple blood transfusion, which can often be given when you are an out-patient. An alternative might be injections of a drug called epoetin (Eprex, or NeoRecormon), which stimulates the bone marrow to make new red blood cells. In the last year or two, doctors have discovered that even very mild levels of anaemia, which would not normally be troublesome, can lead to severe tiredness in people who are having chemotherapy, and correcting this can make a big difference to how they feel. Similarly, giving antibiotics, or antifungal drugs, for an infection, or analgesics to relieve pain, or prescribing antidepressants for people who are clinically depressed, can ease the feeling of tiredness quite dramatically.

But often fatigue is simply due to the effects of chemotherapy, and when this is the case it is a matter of adjusting to cope with the situation. A few tips to help with this are:

- Don't feel worried or, worse still, guilty. Severe tiredness during chemotherapy is quite natural, and is something most people experience as part of their treatment. It is not your fault; it is the normal response of your body to all that is going on.
- Prioritize your activities: do the things you have to do – like washing yourself or cleaning your teeth – but try to organize other people to do things like shopping, or helping with the cooking.
- Plan your day: keep a diary so you can see when you are likely to feel most tired – to help you plan rests – and to see which things make you feel more tired, so you can avoid them. Try to plan as few trips up and down the stairs as possible.
- Take regular rests, or cat-naps. If you feel you need to stop and put your feet up, then do so; don't push yourself to carry on.
- Make sure you sleep well at night – a warm bath and a hot milky drink at bedtime will often help, but if sleeping is a problem then let your doctors know and they may prescribe sleeping tablets to help.
- Avoid extremes of temperature: getting over-hot or feeling cold can be tiring.

- Eat healthily, with plenty of fresh fruit and vegetables, and drink at least 2 litres (4 pints) of fluid every day.
- Find things to distract you and take your mind off the tiredness: listening to pleasant music or relaxation tapes, watching daytime television, getting friends to take you out for a drive can all help (often activities that you would normally find trivial or boring can be much more entertaining and absorbing when you are tired).
- Try some gentle exercise. Although it may sound strange, there is good evidence that gentle exercise can often reduce fatigue. This is not to say that you should sign up for the gym and attempt vigorous work-outs, but, if you can manage it, a stroll round the neighbourhood for 20 to 30 minutes, five or six times a week, might make a big difference to how you feel.

Even when your course of chemotherapy is over, tiredness is likely to last for some time afterwards, certainly for several months. Generally speaking, the older you are, the longer it takes to recover your stamina; and if you have radiotherapy as well as chemotherapy, then this can slow your return to normal energy levels. Studies suggest that even a year after treatment has finished, about one in five people will still regularly have days when they feel fatigued. So don't be worried if your lack of energy doesn't improve immediately, and allow for this in planning your life and activities after chemotherapy.

Mouth problems

Chemotherapy can affect your mouth in several ways. Sometimes it can cause a sore mouth. If this happens, it usually comes on a few days after you have had your treatment. When you look in your mouth there may be nothing to see, or there may be some redness of the lining of your mouth (the mucosa), and sometimes there may be small ulcers. This inflammation and soreness of the lining of the mouth is called mucositis.

If your blood count is on the low side, or if you are on steroids or antibiotics, or if you are very run down, you may also get an infection in your mouth. The most common type of infection is called thrush (also known as *oral candidiasis*, or *oral monilia*). This usually shows up as small whitish patches on the mucosa and the surface of the tongue. Another quite common problem with chemotherapy is getting a dry mouth, and this can also lead to changes of taste, with some foods, and drinks, tasting different from normal.

One drug that is particularly associated with oral mucositis is methotrexate. If this problem develops, then giving a short course of folinic acid (leucovorin) tablets for a day or two can help, and giving the tablets after subsequent courses of the drug greatly reduces the risk of any further mouth soreness.

A sore mouth

The chances of getting a sore mouth do vary depending on your treatment; some drugs, or combinations of drugs, are more likely to cause mucositis than others. Usually your doctors or nurses will warn you if oral soreness is likely to happen, but if they don't mention it, then you can always ask them about it. If it has been flagged up as a possible side effect, there are a number of things you can do that will help reduce the chances of it developing. These include:

- Having a routine check-up with your dentist before you start treatment, just to be sure there are no obvious tooth or gum problems that need to be dealt with before your chemotherapy.
- Sucking crushed ice for 15 to 30 minutes before your chemotherapy is given, and continuing this while you are having the drugs and for about half an hour afterwards, can sometimes prevent mouth soreness. Check with your chemotherapy nurses whether this might be a good idea in your case.
- Maintaining good oral hygiene; this means cleaning your teeth at least twice a day. Using a normal toothbrush can be uncomfortable, so using a soft toothbrush, or a child's brush, might help. You may find that your usual toothpaste makes your mouth and gums sore, and changing to a brand for 'sensitive teeth', like Sensodyne Original or Macleans Sensitive, might help. Mouthwashes can also be useful, and you can try these if you find that brushing your teeth is really painful. There are preparations you can get from your chemist or supermarket that help to prevent infection; these include chlorhexidine, Corsodyl, and thymol. For simply keeping your mouth clean you can make your own mouthwash with a teaspoonful of baking powder (sodium bicarbonate) dissolved in a glass of warm water, and use this to rinse out your mouth thoroughly morning and night.
- Keeping your mouth moist is a good idea, and some tips on how

to do this are given below in the section called 'A dry mouth'.
- Changing your diet. There are some foods and drinks that can make your mouth sore if the mucosa is sensitive. These include very hot and spicy foods, vinegar, salt, neat spirits (whisky, brandy, gin, etc.) and acid drinks like grapefruit juice and some types of orange juice – so avoiding these might be a good idea.

If you get a sore mouth, then do mention it to your nurses or doctors. They will be able to check for signs of infection and give you advice on what to do. If you have got thrush, then this is easily treated by a course of an antifungal drug like nystatin, or amphotericin, for a few days. These drugs are given either as a pastille to suck four times a day, or as a mouthwash that you rinse round your mouth and then swallow four times a day. If there is no evidence of infection, then some of the other things you can do to help a sore mouth after your chemotherapy include:

- Using a painkilling mouthwash. Difflam Oral Rinse is a mouthwash you can buy over the counter which can help. It is also available as a spray. Some people find using the full-strength mouthwash stings, and diluting it with an equal amount of warm water may help. An alternative is to make your own mouthwash using soluble aspirin, dissolving a couple of tablets in a glass of warm water and using this to rinse your mouth well three or four times a day.
- If you actually have mouth ulcers, then there is a wide range of gels, pastes and sprays that you can get that might help. These include Bonjela gel, Biora gel, Medijel, Rinstead contact pastilles, and many more. Your local pharmacist will always be able to advise you on what is available.
- Sometimes taking a mild painkiller can be helpful. Paracetamol capsules, or soluble paracetamol tablets, taken two or three times daily, may reduce your discomfort.

Usually the mucositis associated with chemotherapy only lasts a few days and will have disappeared completely within a week or so.

A dry mouth

If you get a dry mouth during your treatment, there are a number of things that might help. These include:

- Keeping your mouth moist with regular fluids. You should be drinking at least 2 litres (4 pints) of fluid every day during your treatment, but supplementing this with regular sips of water or other soft drinks can help (fizzy water, or fizzy drinks, tend to be better than still fluids). Sucking ice cubes or crushed ice is another idea.

- Smearing the surface of your tongue and the lining of your mouth with a little olive oil or melted butter will keep things moist for a while and is often particularly effective last thing at night.
- Chewing sugar-free chewing gum, or sugar-free fruit pastilles, can help stimulate your salivary glands to make moisture for your mouth. In the same way, sucking pineapple chunks may help.
- Cleaning your mouth regularly with baking powder (sodium bicarbonate) mouthwashes (one teaspoonful of powder in a glass of warm water) keeps the mucosa moist and clean.
- Drinking a glass of sherry (especially dry, rather than medium or sweet sherry) about a quarter of an hour before a meal can often stimulate the salivary glands, and your digestive system, to make eating easier and more appealing.
- Moistening your food helps, using plenty of gravy or sauces. On the other hand, dry foods are best avoided, especially things like crackers, flaky pastry and chocolate, which all tend to stick to the lining of your mouth.
- There are a number of over-the-counter preparations of artificial saliva that some people find useful. These may come as sprays, gels, pastilles or tablets, and include Saliva Orthana, Glandosane, Luborant, Saliveze, Salivix and SST. Once again, your local pharmacist will be happy to advise you what is available.
- Using a lip balm to moisten your lips and keep them soft might make a difference.
- There are also some things to try to avoid. Smoking, alcohol and caffeine (in tea and coffee) all tend to make your mouth dry, so cutting back on these is a good thing.

Hair loss

As I mentioned earlier, hair loss is a major worry for many people when they are first told they need chemotherapy. The likelihood of losing your hair varies greatly with different chemotherapy treatments. With some drugs, hair loss (alopecia) hardly ever occurs, while with others it is almost inevitable. When alopecia does occur, it may be anything from some thinning of the hair of the head to complete loss of all body hair.

Some general tips to help protect your hair when you are going to have chemotherapy are:

- Avoid using heated products like curling tongs or heated rollers.
- Try to wash your hair less often. The fewer times you wash your hair the better (but obviously you will have to find your own balance between reducing the frequency of washes and what you feel comfortable with).
- Avoid shampoos and conditioners with lots of chemicals: try using a baby shampoo.
- Avoid hair dyes and colourants, unless they are completely organic (plant-based), with no added chemicals.
- Avoid perms.
- If you have very long hair, then having it cut to a shorter style may help.

If your treatment does involve drugs that carry a high risk of alopecia, the one thing that can sometimes be done to try to prevent, or reduce, this is scalp cooling. There are various types of scalp cooling, but the general principle is to chill the scalp, usually by wearing a special padded hat that contains a gel. The hat is stored in a freezer and is then strapped firmly on your head about half an hour before you are due to have your drugs.

You carry on wearing the hat while the drugs are given and for about half an hour afterwards. If your drugs are being given over more than a few minutes, you may need to have your hat changed to make sure your scalp remains chilled.

The idea behind this is that keeping the scalp very cold makes the blood vessels in the skin of your head contract, so the blood supply to the hair follicles is reduced and they will be less affected by the circulating chemotherapy drugs.

Scalp cooling doesn't always work. For many people it will prevent or greatly reduce the amount of hair loss, but for others it has very little effect. Some people find scalp cooling uncomfortable. The hat is very cold, and can often cause headaches, so it does not suit everyone. Scalp cooling only helps to preserve the hair on your head; it won't stop hair loss anywhere else.

If you do develop alopecia, then your chemotherapy team will give you advice on ways of coping with this. The most obvious of these is having a wig. These can be supplied by the NHS. Most Chemotherapy Units have a specially trained member of staff who can discuss the options with you and arrange a wig that meets the colour and style you would like. There is a cost for this: the standard NHS charge is about £50, but if you are exempt from normal prescription charges, you won't have to pay this. Many Chemotherapy Units have ways of helping with the costs. Alternatives to wigs include headscarves and bandanas, which allow some people to turn their hair loss into a fashion statement!

A small bonus is that some men find that while they are having chemotherapy they don't need to shave.

It is important to remember that if you develop alopecia it will always be temporary. However much hair you lose, it will grow back again within a few months of completing your chemotherapy – although it does often come back with a different colour and texture, often being curly or wavy, with a 'pepper and salt' colouring and slightly thicker, coarser texture.

Fertility

Chemotherapy can affect fertility for both men and women, but the risk of becoming infertile varies greatly with different treatments. After some types of chemotherapy, sterility is inevitable; after others it is almost unknown. So if you are thinking that you might want to have children in the future, do discuss this with your doctors before you start treatment, so that they can work out the treatment that is least likely to interfere with your fertility, while still being effective against the cancer.

If there is still a likelihood that treatment will make you sterile, there is really nothing you can do in terms of lifestyle changes (diet, exercise and so on) that will reduce this risk. There are, however, other measures that may help. These are different for men and women.

For men, if there is a chance that treatment will affect your fertility, you should always be offered the chance of sperm banking before you begin chemotherapy. This involves giving several samples of your sperm, which are then frozen and stored. Sometimes the presence of the cancer actually reduces the number and quality of your sperm, but, even so, having your sperm stored is still worthwhile, as it may still be possible to use it to produce a pregnancy in the future, although success cannot be guaranteed. Incidentally, not having sex for a couple of days before you give the sperm samples will increase the quality of your specimen. Unfortunately, freezing the sample does further reduce the quality of the sperm, but once they are frozen they can be kept indefinitely without any further deterioration. When you and your partner are finally ready to contemplate having children, your sperm can be thawed and used (this will involve some form of artificial insemination of your partner). The rules vary from hospital to hospital, but you may find that there is a charge for the storage of your sperm.

For women, the options are more limited. Freezing and storage of embryos that can be thawed and reimplanted into the womb after treatment is possible, but delaying your treatment long enough for this to be arranged will not usually be advisable. Even if you do go through this process, the chances of a successful pregnancy are probably still only about one in five. Having an operation to take away eggs (oocytes) from the ovary and have these frozen, or taking away pieces of ovarian tissue for storage (that could be replaced after treatment to try and make the ovaries work again), are both possible, but are really experimental approaches that are still being developed, with, at the moment, very little chance of success. Another option that you could consider is egg donation, where, after your treatment is over, your womb could be implanted with eggs donated by another woman. This has resulted in successful pregnancies for some women after their ovaries have failed as a result of chemotherapy.

Many types of chemotherapy will reduce fertility – lowering sperm counts in men, or stopping the periods in women – while you are actually having treatment, but will not result in permanent infertility. But it may take anywhere from six months to two years for your testicular, or ovarian, function to get back to normal. Usually, though, doctors would advise against having children in the first year after your treatment, so this possible delay should not be too much of a problem.

If your fertility is reduced, but returns after chemotherapy, or if it was unaffected by treatment, the drugs that you have had will not lead to any increase in the chances of birth defects in children that you may father, or give birth to, in the future. So it will be perfectly safe to have children as soon as your doctors think it is OK from the point of view of your cancer and its treatment.

7

Other ways to help

In this chapter we will look at some more general ways of helping you to cope with chemotherapy.

The spiritual dimension

For many people their religious faith can give valuable support during the stresses and strains of cancer treatment. This spiritual dimension often provides comfort and reassurance, and gives emotional strength to work through the more difficult days. Prayer and belief can offer hope and meaning when times are bad.

This is a very personal subject, and the beliefs that each of us hold will vary in their nature, and in their importance to us. But one general point to make is that, like everything else we will discuss in this chapter, your faith should be used as a means of support during your chemotherapy, and not as an alternative to it. Spiritual strength can make living with the effects of chemotherapy easier, and it may even increase the chances of successful treatment, but it cannot take the place of conventional medicine: the two should always work together.

Talking

Talking can be very helpful, although that does not mean it is always easy.

Speaking about your treatment, and your cancer, can have many benefits. Sharing your experience, your concerns, your worries, your problems, can be very positive. That is not to say that other people will always have answers, although sometimes they might, but simply expressing your feelings can help. It can help because it lets you begin to work out what your worries are, what things you need to know or do, what questions you need to ask, what support you might need. Just explaining things that may be troubling you can often make them less troubling, and sometimes reassure you that your fears are unnecessary, or that something you thought would be a major issue in your case is unlikely to happen, or can be handled relatively easily.

Talking also helps you to get a sense of control over your situation. It helps you to sort out what things are important to you personally, both positively – things you want to do and achieve, and negatively – things that you are worried might happen. You can then decide which of these things is important, and begin to plan how to do the things you want to do, and how to find out about, and cope with, the things that are causing you concern.

Bottling things up, or keeping things to yourself, can often make matters worse. When thoughts go round and round in our heads, our fears can often get out of proportion, and then the worry just goes on growing. But by sharing your anxieties, bringing things out into the open, that vicious circle can often be broken; and although the basic problem may not go away, it can be a whole lot easier to live with.

Sometimes just explaining things and being reassured that the feelings you have are quite natural in your situation can be reassuring in itself. Knowing that your sensations and emotions are normal, and understandable in the circumstances, can be a relief.

Of course, there is always the question of who to talk to. A caring and sympathetic partner is the obvious choice: someone who knows you, and cares deeply about your well-being, and who, even if they cannot change things, can listen with understanding, and appreciate how you are feeling. But not everyone has such a partner, or you may feel that talking in this way is placing too great a burden on them (although very often these sorts of conversations can actually deepen the bonds that form a relationship and bring you even closer).

But if talking to your nearest and dearest is something you find difficult, then it may be easier to talk to someone on your medical team. The people you are likely to see most of during your treatment are your chemotherapy nurses, and it is likely that you will get to know one or two of them very well during this time. If you ask, they will often be able to find time to chat about your worries with you and, once again, may often be able to reassure you that things you are frightened of are unlikely to happen, or give you good advice on how to reduce the risk of them happening – or how to cope with them if they do.

Some hospital departments have counsellors available whom you can talk to about your illness, your treatment, and all the emotional and practical concerns that it is causing. Another alternative that is sometimes possible is to ask to meet and talk to other people who have had your type of cancer, and had similar treatment, to see how they got on and how they managed the sort of issues you are having to face. In many places this sort of opportunity is offered by cancer support groups (see p. 67), where people (and their relatives and carers) who have, or have had, cancer can meet on a regular basis to talk about their experiences. Discovering that other people have had similar thoughts and fears to yours, and realizing that the issues you are facing are not something you have to confront alone but can share with others and sometimes learn from their experience, can often be very comforting.

Although these sorts of exchanges can sometimes be very valuable, it is important to remember that each of us is a unique individual, and that even when someone has had the same type of cancer as you, and had treatment that may have been nearly the same as yours, their experience of things, the side effects they might have had, their feelings about everything that was going on, their worries, and the solutions they found, may be very different to your own experience, so do not expect that everything that happened to them will happen to you in the same way.

If you do want to talk about things, let people know. Very often, family and friends will be worried that asking you about your condition, and how you are feeling and how things are going, will upset you, so will often think that by not talking about what is going on they will be doing you a kindness, and sparing you distress. So if you want to talk about your treatment, or your cancer, do not hesitate to bring the subject up. Bringing things out into the open will often make for a much more relaxed and easy atmosphere all round among those who are close to you.

Equally, if there are times when you don't want to talk, when you just want a bit of peace, or when going over things again will all be a bit too much, then say so. Let people know when you need some time to yourself, to get your thoughts in order, or just to mentally get away from it all for a while. You are in control, so take control and talk as much, or as little, as you want to.

Diet: what to eat

There is a huge amount of information and misinformation about diet and cancer. Every week, stories appear in the newspapers, in magazines, and on the television about this or that food, which is either good or bad, and there are countless suggestions for diets that will help prevent or fight the disease.

In trying to make sense of all this confusing, and often conflicting, advice, the first step is to realize that there are two completely separate questions when it comes to the subject of food and cancer. The first is, can what we eat increase, or reduce, our risk of getting cancer? The second is, once someone has cancer, can their diet increase their chances of being cured?

There is now good scientific evidence that what people eat does alter their chances of getting some types of cancer. For example, a high consumption of red meat increases the risk of getting two of the most common types of cancer: bowel cancer and prostate cancer. On the other hand, there are many myths about diet and cancer risk. For instance, there is a popular belief that a high intake of dairy products increases the risk of getting breast cancer, but there is no real evidence for this (although being overweight does increase a woman's chances of getting the disease). On the positive side, there are also foods that can help to reduce the likelihood of cancer: a diet rich in fibre (with plenty of fruit and vegetables) makes bowel cancer less likely; and eating plenty of fish and tomato products is linked to a lower risk of prostate cancer.

But these things all relate to preventing or avoiding getting cancer in the first place. It is thought, for example, that the harmful foods that are linked to cancer development will, over a period of time, help to trigger changes in the cells to make them cancerous. But once that change has taken place, and the cancer has begun to grow, there is virtually no evidence that a change in diet can slow down, or reverse, the progression of the cancer. So once someone actually has a cancer, changing their diet is not likely to influence how rapidly, or slowly, the tumour grows, and is not going to make any difference to whether or not they will be cured.

Despite this, there are countless recommendations given in the media, on websites, at independent non-NHS clinics, and by well-meaning people everywhere, for diets that will help to cure the cancer. Many people believe passionately in these, and are convinced of their benefits, but none of these diets has been shown scientifically to alter how a cancer will behave.

So when you are having chemotherapy, what you eat will make no difference to the chances of success of your treatment. It is very necessary to remember this, so that you can focus on what is really important about your diet during this time.

The two main things that are important about what you eat during chemotherapy are that you have what you enjoy, and are comfortable with, and that you try to keep a healthy balance in your food.

When it comes to enjoying, and being comfortable with, what you eat there are a number of things to remember. These include:

- It is quite likely that your tastes will change while you are going through chemotherapy. Some things you were fond of before may taste different, and even unpleasant, whereas things you didn't particularly like now seem very tasty. So be prepared to vary your diet.
- Your appetite will vary a lot while you are having treatment and it is likely that there will be times when you won't really fancy food. Generally speaking, having light meals, or snacks, and eating little and often, is easier and more pleasant than having one or two big meals a day.
- Well-meaning relatives and friends are likely to get anxious if they see you are eating less, especially if you start to lose a bit of weight. But having people continually coaxing and encouraging you to have something can be very off-putting, and make you feel even less like eating. As long as you are drinking plenty, then having the odd day or two when you don't eat very much is quite all right.
- Your system will probably cope best with foods that are easy to digest. So changing from red meats to things like chicken, eggs or fish, and avoiding heavy puddings, fatty pastries and rich sauces, can all help. But if you do suddenly fancy something rich and stodgy, then go for it – eat what you enjoy.
- Although most people do lose weight when they are having chemotherapy, quite a few find that they actually start to put on weight. The combination of taking less exercise, having short courses of steroids (which may stimulate the appetite), and sometimes comfort eating, can all contribute to this. Putting on a few pounds (or a kilogram or two) is not usually a worry, but if you find your weight is really going up, then have a word with your chemotherapy nurses to get a bit of advice about your diet.

For a healthy diet, fresh fruit and vegetables and plenty of fluids are important. Some of the 'cancer diets' that you may come across recommend ridiculous amounts of certain things – at least 500 grams (1 pound 2 ounces) of grated raw carrot every day, or masses of lightly steamed broccoli, or limitless quantities of raw blueberries, for example. Don't be dictated to by these recommendations; so long as you are eating a selection of fresh fruit and vegetables on a regular basis, this is what matters. Aiming for the Department of Health's target of five portions of fruit or veg every day is a good target but, once again, if you don't feel up to it then don't force yourself.

As far as fluid is concerned, it's worth stressing again that you should try to aim for at least 2 litres (4 pints) every day. Plenty of water is good to keep the system flushed through, but any other drinks you fancy are OK.

Incidentally, many people worry about having alcohol while they are on chemotherapy. Certainly getting drunk is not a good idea, but, except in rare circumstances, having a glass of wine or a pint of beer will not do you any harm at all. In fact, alcohol can sometimes help if your appetite is poor: a glass of sherry, and particularly dry sherry, about 15 minutes before you are due to eat can often stimulate the digestion and make food more appealing.

Most Chemotherapy Units have specially trained dieticians who work with them. So if during your treatment you are worried about what you should eat and drink, or if you find you are losing, or putting on, more weight than you are comfortable with, do ask to have a word with them so that you can get expert professional advice.

Exercise

We are constantly being told that regular exercise is good for us, and this is true. But when you are having chemotherapy you will often feel worn out, and probably not very well, and the thought of rushing off to the gym, or going for a quick jog round the block, is unlikely to be high on your list of priorities.

Exercise can make you feel better, though. It helps fight off depression, it can improve your appetite, and reduce the risk of constipation. It lowers your chances of getting blood clots in your veins (thrombosis) and is a way of taking your mind off things for a while – a distraction from everything else that is going on.

The secret of exercise during chemotherapy is all down to personal balance. Trying to force yourself to do vigorous activities that you really don't feel you can face is just as bad as simply retreating to bed and giving up. The key word to go with 'exercise' in this situation is 'gentle'. Do enough to keep your body mobile and in reasonable shape. Keep in trim by basing your activities on what you did before you started the treatment. If you used to run ten miles a day, in training for the half-marathon, then cut back to a regular trot round the park; if all you managed was four trips up and down stairs each day, then still try to make that short journey a couple of times a day. Don't push yourself unduly, don't try and take on strenuous new activities because you feel you have to, but equally don't stop everything.

It is often said that walking is the best exercise, and this is probably true during your treatment. If you can manage a short walk, stroll or amble about each day, this will keep your system ticking over, and can also provide a period of time when you can get out of the house and have a bit of a change of scene.

Complementary therapies

Complementary therapies can be used alongside conventional treatments, like surgery, radiotherapy or chemotherapy, to help people cope with their illness. They are not intended to cure the cancer, but are used to ease any side effects of treatment, and improve general well-being.

They are different from alternative therapies, which are unconventional treatments given to try to control or cure the cancer. Various claims have been made that alternative therapies work, but there is no medical proof that they do. Sometimes the alternative therapies concerned have actually been shown to be ineffective, or even harmful, but they are still being promoted to unsuspecting members of the public. These therapies frequently involve considerable expense, and practitioners may insist on demanding changes in lifestyle, with outlandish diets, or special supplements of 'essential elements', 'vital vitamins', or 'immunity-boosting drugs' – none of which has been scientifically proven to work.

This contrasts with many complementary therapies, which are generally used alongside mainstream medical care, and which are safe, well understood, can actually be pleasant to undergo, and usually have a positive effect on well-being.

While health professionals remain highly unconvinced by the claims made by the advocates of alternative therapies, their attitude to complementary therapies has changed greatly over the last ten years, with more and more doctors and nurses seeing them as useful additions to conventional therapies that can very often improve the quality of life of their patients. Combining conventional and complementary therapy can frequently be a productive partnership.

Many people try complementary therapies while they are having chemotherapy. The main types of complementary therapies are the touch therapies (aromatherapy, massage therapy, reflexology, and acupuncture), fitness and movement therapies (yoga, t'ai chi, and qigong), psychological therapies (relaxation, meditation, visualization, music therapy) and dietary therapies.

Touch therapies

Aromatherapy involves the use of essential oils. These are plant extracts that have distinctive smells. Each of the different essential oils is believed to have particular physical or psychological effects – for example, lavender and eucalyptus help to ease stress, while camomile reduces inflammation. The oils may be used in massage, or given as inhalations, aromatic baths, or applied as creams or lotions. Reflexology is a type of foot massage. It is based on the belief that areas on the feet match different parts of the body, and that by applying pressure to these areas energy paths are activated that can produce beneficial effects. Acupuncture is based on ancient Chinese medicine, which believes that the body's energy, or chi, moves in pathways, or meridians, beneath the skin, and by inserting needles into these meridians a healing response can be stimulated.

Aromatherapy and reflexology are very relaxing, and many people with cancer say that they feel better after having these treatments. Acupuncture is rather more uncomfortable, but there is some evidence that it can help ease pain and sickness if these are a problem.

With these different therapies, there is at the present time very little scientific evidence for their value, although an increasing number of clinical trials using these treatments are under way, and there is a growing belief that they can be helpful.

Fitness and movement therapies

These involve more active participation, rather than just lying back and enjoying the therapy, but many people find that they help to ease anxiety and depression, as well as giving a bit of gentle exercise to keep up overall fitness.

Psychological therapies

These can be as simple as just relaxing in a quiet room listening to restful music, or might involve working with a counsellor who teaches you relaxation techniques, or uses visualization (picturing your body and how it is working to fight the cancer, or reduce the side effects of treatment). Art therapy and music therapy – using drawing or painting to channel your emotions, or listening to (and sometimes taking part in) live music performances – are other types of psychological therapy. Many people find that these techniques can help to ease stress and anxiety and make them feel better during their treatment.

Dietary changes

These may involve simply taking one or more supplements to your normal diet, or a complete change in the way you eat. This is one area where the boundaries between complementary and alternative therapies do become blurred. There are many people who claim that particular diets or supplements will help ease side effects of treatment, and sometimes suggest that they will actually help to control the cancer or stop it coming back. Very often these claims are based on the belief that this change in diet will boost the immune system. Unfortunately, there is virtually no evidence for any of these claims. Also, occasionally these diets can be quite extreme, and unpleasant (or expensive), and actually reduce your quality of life rather than enhancing it. Having a normal balanced range of foods, with plenty of fresh fruit and vegetables, is very hard to beat.

Complementary therapies have a lot of appeal. They often lead to emotional and spiritual well-being, with a relief of stress and anxiety, and they may actually reduce some of the side effects of treatment, or make them easier to live with. They also offer some empowerment. This is one part of your treatment, and overall care, that you can take control of and decide exactly how and when you want to use it. Furthermore, at a time when – following the diagnosis of cancer and all the tests and treatments that follow on from that – it can seem that the running of everyday life has gone completely out of your own hands, having something where you make the decisions can be very valuable.

Each of us is different, and with complementary therapies people vary greatly in their responses. How much these therapies will help in coping with the stresses and strains of chemotherapy, and how much they will relieve any side effects like tiredness or sickness, varies hugely from one person to another: some people will feel a real benefit, whereas others won't notice any difference. If you want to try any of these therapies, do check first with your medical team that it is all right for you to do so, and then give it a try. If you find that you enjoy it and feel better for it, then that is great, but if it doesn't help, then don't hesitate to stop. Sometimes, particularly with diets, people start on a new regime and find that they really don't like it but feel they must continue or they will get worse. This is not what complementary therapies are about – they are there to improve your quality of life, not reduce it, and if you do try a new diet, or any other type of complementary therapy, and find that you feel more miserable as a result, then do stop it at once.

Times are changing, and conventional doctors are becoming more sympathetic towards complementary therapies, and some Cancer Centres will offer these as part of their service to NHS patients. But unfortunately the availability of these services in hospitals, or at GPs' surgeries, is still very patchy and variable, and the likelihood is that if you do want to pursue any of these options, then you will have to make your own arrangements and pay for them.

Information

For many people, simply understanding what is going on, what is happening to them, is a very important part of being able to cope with difficult experiences such as having cancer and undergoing chemotherapy. That means knowledge, and that means seeking information.

Your doctors and nurses should keep you fully informed of everything about your illness and its treatment, but sometimes they don't, and even when they do there may be things you want to know more about.

Information comes in many different forms – the simple chat with your medical team can be very helpful, but leaves you with nothing to refer to afterwards. Therefore, more and more often nowadays these conversations are being backed up by leaflets, booklets, video cassettes or DVDs that you can take away and look at afterwards. Then there are books (like this one!) and, of course, the internet.

There is a vast amount of information out there, dealing with every aspect of cancer and its treatment that you could possibly think of. The two problems are getting hold of that information, and knowing whether or not it is reliable. The Department of Health is very keen for people with cancer to have as much information as they want, so your medical team should welcome any questions you have about where to get this, and be able to point you in the right direction. They may offer leaflets, or booklets that they have produced themselves, or provide literature from approved organizations such as CancerBACUP, Macmillan Cancer Relief, or Cancer Research UK. They can also give you the contact details to reach these organizations' websites, where there is a wealth of information. More details about this are given in 'Useful addresses' at the back of this book. You are perfectly free to get in touch with any of these groups yourself, and do not need the prior approval of your doctors.

Going down this route is probably far safer than a simple internet search. Although there is limitless good and reliable coverage of all aspects of cancer on the internet, there is also a huge amount of misinformation, some of which is not only misleading, but downright dangerous – just because something is on the internet does not mean it can be believed, even though it may look and sound very convincing.

Cancer support groups

Another source of both support and information can be a local cancer support group. These developed informally during the 1980s and have grown in number since then. They have no fixed pattern, and so vary very much from place to place. Sometimes they are run by specialist nurses from the hospital (in which case they often focus on one particular type of cancer), or they may be based in the community, associated with, for example, a local health centre, a church, or a community centre. What the various groups do have in common is the opportunity to meet other people in a similar situation to yourself, or who have been through the same sort of experience in the past, so that you can compare and contrast your views and theirs in a social setting.

There is often some form of professional input in these groups, with informal talks from experts in various fields on one or other aspect of the subject, and there is likely to be a supply of suitable background information, or someone who can give advice on where to get such information. There may also be other activities, like the availability of some complementary therapies, or access to spiritual support from local faith leaders.

The availability of cancer support groups, and the format of the groups, differs from place to place, but if the idea interests you, then do ask your doctors and nurses about it, and they should be able to let you know what is on offer in your area.

8

Chemotherapy and everyday life

Although it may change, your everyday life does not stop while you are having chemotherapy. Work, holidays, money, sex, friends and neighbours are all parts of day-to-day living that might be affected by your treatment. This chapter looks at some of the problems you might meet, and offers some advice to help you cope with them.

Work and chemotherapy

The effect of chemotherapy on someone's lifestyle will depend on the type of treatment they need, and their individual reactions to that treatment. For a few people, chemotherapy will have little or no impact on their day-to-day lives; for others, who need intensive treatment over a long period, their lives will change completely.

A typical course of chemotherapy will involve treatment over four to six months. Even if you have few obviously troublesome side effects during this time, it is likely that the treatment will make you feel more tired than usual. You are also likely to have lots of visits to the hospital, not only for the chemotherapy itself, but also for blood tests and check-ups. Once the chemotherapy has actually finished, it is quite likely that the feeling of fatigue will last for some months afterwards.

These various disruptions caused by the treatment do mean that continuing to work while having chemotherapy is very difficult for most people. So if you are working, and facing the prospect of having chemotherapy, then you need to think ahead about how this will affect your job.

In order to help your planning you will need to know some basic facts about your cancer and its treatment. So you should ask your doctors and nurses some of the following questions:

- How long will the chemotherapy go on for?
- What will be involved, in terms of the number and frequency of hospital visits?
- What are the likely side effects, how troublesome might they be, and how long are they going to last?

- What is the likely outcome of the treatment: will your cancer probably be cured completely, or is the chemotherapy being given to try and control it for a period of time before it comes back again?

And, of course, you can get their advice on how easy, or difficult, they feel it might be for you to carry on working during treatment.

Once you have got this information you can start to think about what you personally would like to do with respect to your job. For some people, work is the most important thing in their lives and they would do anything possible to avoid having time off. For others, work is a drudge and a chore, and the chance to give it up, even for a while, would be a real bonus. Also, for some people, the diagnosis of cancer, and its treatment, might give them the opportunity for early retirement, or retirement on the grounds of ill health, and this may be something else you might want to think about.

When you have got an idea of how you would like to handle your working life during, and immediately after, chemotherapy, the next thing is to talk to your employer about the options available. Most employers will be sympathetic in this situation, and try and make arrangements for things like time off, flexible working hours, lighter duties, or working from home. If your workplace has an occupational health department, or a human resources team, then chatting to them can often give you a good idea of the choices open to you. They will be able to tell you about your company's sickness policies and your entitlements to sick leave and pay during that time. They will also treat their discussions with you in strict confidence.

Most employers are very supportive of staff who develop cancer and need chemotherapy. But if you do have problems, then you do also have rights. Most people with cancer will be covered by the Disability Discrimination Act. This Act says that it is unlawful for an employer to discriminate against a person because of their disability. To be classed as 'disabled' under the Act, someone with cancer must have symptoms, or side effects of treatment, that interfere with their day-to-day activities; so if the effects of your chemotherapy mean that your treatment will limit, or prevent, your ability to work, then you should be covered. The Act also covers people who have recovered from a disability, so if you have been cured as a result of your treatment, your employer cannot discriminate against you because you have had cancer in the past.

Under the terms of the Act, an employer should make 'reasonable adjustments' to workplaces and working practices to make sure that you are not at any substantial disadvantage compared to your colleagues at work. The phrase 'reasonable adjustments' would usually cover things like time off for hospital visits, changes in your working hours, avoiding physically demanding jobs, or allowing a gradual return to work after a period of sick leave.

If you feel your supervisors, or managers, are being unreasonable or unhelpful, then you could talk to your occupational health, or human resources, team at work. If you need advice outside of your workplace, then you could talk to your union representative, or contact your local Citizens Advice Bureau. Very occasionally, it may even help to get guidance from a lawyer.

Holidays and travel

The fact that most chemotherapy treatments are given every few weeks means that it is sometimes possible to go away for a short holiday between courses. If you are thinking of taking a short break somewhere in Britain, this is usually fairly straightforward, but a holiday abroad may be more difficult.

For a trip within the UK, the first thing to do is to check with your doctors and nurses that they think it will be safe for you to do this, and it won't interfere with any treatment or tests that you need. Once you have their agreement, then the two things you need to make sure of are that you take a good supply of all the medicines you need, or might need, with you and that you have some written information about your cancer and its treatment. This is a wise precaution, because if you were to be taken ill, and had difficulty in getting straight back to your own hospital, then the doctors where you were staying would need to have details about your condition and the drugs you were having, so they could take care of you. These days, most people having chemotherapy will have their own 'handheld record' books, giving all the necessary information and contact details, so taking this with you would be the ideal. If you don't have your own record book, then ask your doctor or nurses for a letter that gives all the relevant information to take with you.

Holidays abroad present more problems. Even if your medical team are happy for you to travel overseas you may have difficulty in getting travel insurance. Most insurers will be reluctant to issue cover to people who are having chemotherapy, or who are within a month or so of having completed their treatment. Some insurers also refuse cover if you have recently had a blood transfusion. It is worth shopping around, however, because companies do vary and you may find that you can get cover, although you may have to pay a premium, and they might also want a report from your doctor confirming that it is all right for you to go abroad.

Getting insurance is often easier if you are travelling to countries within the EU, or certain other countries that have reciprocal health agreements with the UK, which means that any treatment you have there would either be free or relatively cheap. By contrast, countries where health costs are much higher, like the USA, can be more difficult to get insurance for.

If you are going abroad, even if you have got insurance, there are a few other things to bear in mind:

- As with trips within the UK, taking written details of your cancer and its treatment is essential.
- Do take a good supply of all the drugs you need (and take some extra in case of delays on your journey). If you have drugs that have to be given by injection, using needles and syringes, or if you are taking narcotic drugs, like morphine, then you may need special permission from the immigration services of the place you are going to, and special documents from your own doctors. Your travel company should be able to advise you, or you could contact the embassy of the country you are hoping to visit.
- Many people with cancer have a higher than normal risk of deep vein thrombosis, and this risk is further increased if you are on certain drugs, like tamoxifen. So if you are going on a long haul flight, check with your doctors to see whether they feel you are at risk, and what precautions you ought to take.
- If you are hoping to go somewhere where you need vaccinations, this could be a problem. Because of the reduced immunity brought about by chemotherapy, some vaccines might actually be dangerous and others could be ineffective. Once again, have a chat with your doctor if you are going to need vaccinations.

People also wonder about going out in the sun when they are having, or have recently had, chemotherapy. In general, chemotherapy drugs don't increase your risk of sunburn, so it is perfectly all right to go out in the sun provided that you are careful, and make sure you don't get burnt. Simply take the necessary precautions, sun creams, sun block, sun hats and so on, that you would normally take if you were going on holiday to somewhere in the sun.

Financial help

Sometimes being on chemotherapy, and the time you need to recover afterwards, can lead to some financial hardship, and there are a number of state benefits that are on offer to help during this period. They are there for the asking, so do not hesitate to apply if you feel they would help you.

The main benefits are:

- Disability Living Allowance (DLA): This allowance is for anyone under 65 who needs help with their day-to-day care because of their illness. A special category within this allowance is called 'special rules', and this is for anyone who is unlikely to live longer than six months. A 'special rules' payment means you get the highest rate of payment possible, your claim is given priority, and payment is made immediately. Although the 'special rules' do say they are for people with a life expectancy of six months or less, most people who have an advanced (incurable) cancer will find that they are able to get this allowance, even if they live considerably longer than six months. Anyone is entitled to this allowance, regardless of their income or savings, and it is tax-free.
- Attendance Allowance (AA): This allowance is similar to the Disability Living Allowance, but is for people of 65 or over. Like the Disability Living Allowance, the Attendance Allowance is not means-tested and is not taxable.
- Invalid Carer's Allowance (ICA): This is a payment to carers. To qualify you have to be over 16, you must not earn more than £79 a week, and you cannot claim any other benefits. Also, the person you care for must be receiving Attendance Allowance or Disability Living Allowance Care Component.

Other government benefits that may help include: Income Support (if you are aged between 18 and 60 and are working less than 16 hours a week); Working Tax Credit (if you are on a low income); Pension Credit (if you are over 60 and on a low income); and Child Tax Credit if you have dependent children. Also, if you are already claiming Income Support, you may be able to get help with your mortgage repayments if you need this.

Another type of support is the Direct Payment scheme. This gives cash to people who need to employ someone to help with their care. This can include making payments to a close relative, provided that they do not live with you. This scheme is run by your local council-run social services, and is separate from the government benefits, which are paid by the Department of Works and Pensions. So even if you have one of the DWP benefits, you can still contact your local social services department to ask about Direct Payments.

In addition to these various state allowances, the charity Macmillan Cancer Relief does give financial grants to cancer patients who are in need. You can apply for these to cover various living expenses, or for things like a special holiday.

Sex

Sex is a sensitive and very personal subject. This means it is often something that people who are going to have chemotherapy feel shy about discussing with their doctors and nurses. Because it is not talked about very much, people do often worry, so it is important to start by stating a few facts.

First, no one can catch cancer from someone else by having sex with them. So there is no risk that you could pass on your cancer to your partner by carrying on with your normal love life.

Second, having sex does not make the cancer worse, or, if it has already been treated successfully, increase the risk of it coming back.

Third, having sex won't interfere with your chemotherapy. It won't stop the drugs from working, or make them any less effective or increase the risk of side effects.

So sex is safe during chemotherapy. Having said this, most doctors recommend that if you do make love while you are going through the treatment, it is a good idea to use a barrier form of protection, with a condom. There are several reasons for this:

- If you are a woman who has not yet gone through the menopause you could still become pregnant while you are having chemotherapy, even if your periods have stopped as a result of the treatment. So you do still need some form of contraception.

- Although there is no very good evidence for it, many experts believe that small traces of the chemotherapy drugs, or chemicals formed by their breakdown in the body, can find their way into the male semen, or into the female fluids that moisten the vagina, and these could cause soreness or discomfort for your partner.

Another word of caution is that if you are a woman and you have had surgery or radiotherapy to your pelvis as part of your treatment before chemotherapy, then you should check how soon it will be safe for you to restart penetrative sex. Your specialist nurses will usually discuss this with you as part of their care during your treatment.

Although there is no medical reason why you should not continue your normal love life during your treatment, many people simply don't feel like it. This may be due to a number of things, including:

- Tiredness: feeling tired, and completely drained of energy, is the most common of all the side effects of chemotherapy and most people just don't feel like having sex when they feel worn out.
- Other side effects: the chemotherapy may cause other side effects which are upsetting and just make you feel miserable. No one is likely to enjoy sex if they are feeling nauseated.
- Anxiety: being worried about your cancer and its treatment is very understandable, and if you are feeling anxious, then you are likely to be less keen on sex.
- Depression: sometimes natural anxiety tips over into clinical depression, generally feeling low and lacking interest in things, including love making.
- The effects of the cancer: if your cancer is still present then the illness itself may be making you feel unwell and switching off your interest.

Any, or all, of these things may affect your feelings about sex while you are having chemotherapy, and for some time afterwards.

The first, and most important, step in handling this change in your feelings is talking. And the most important person to talk to is your partner. Many people find that talking about sex, and in particular their own needs and emotions, is not easy. But letting your partner know what you are experiencing is essential, so that the two of you can reach a shared understanding of the way you are feeling. Talking may be hard, but it is far better than hiding your worries and concerns, or trying to pretend that things are normal when they are not.

Usually partners will be understanding, supportive and sympathetic. So that once you break the ice of bringing up the subject of sex, finding ways forward together to adapt to your altered desires and emotions should become easier, and you will at least have created a starting point from where you can work together to sort out any problems that your change in sexuality is causing in your relationship.

However, for some couples communication is more difficult, and even just starting to talk together about anything as sensitive as sex may be hard. If this is the case, then counselling may be a help. A trained counsellor might well be able to overcome the reservations, inhibitions or anxieties that are holding back an open discussion of the subject, and not only help sort out what the problems are, but pave the way to finding solutions to them. Quite a few hospitals do have counsellors available for their cancer patients, and there are also sources of help outside the NHS.

Once this background awareness of the situation has been established, you can go on to look at ways of coping with it.

The most likely difficulty is a mismatch in desire, with the person who is having treatment feeling less sexy, while their partner's libido remains much the same. This is very natural for both parties, and neither of you should be guilty about the way you are feeling. Once again, talking helps to reach an understanding that your physical desires are different, and that that difference is entirely reasonable. From that basis of acceptance of difference, you can begin to sort out how to handle the situation. The solutions will be different for different people. They might include an agreed abstinence, a period of celibacy till you both feel the time is right, or you might adjust your relationship to one of hugs, caresses and cuddles, showing your love physically without actual sex; or you might change your approach to sex, with a greater emphasis on things like touching, stroking and masturbation, rather than penetrative sex, or changes in position that make actual intercourse more relaxed and less tiring.

These adjustments can only be made by the two of you, and can only be achieved by talking and understanding. There are no rights and wrongs, no set rules, for how the sexual dynamics of a couple should change at these times, so finding out what works for you is the right answer, rather than thinking there is some magic formula that you ought to try and follow.

There are a few practical issues that are also worth mentioning.

Many women will find that they get vaginal soreness and dryness during their chemotherapy, which can make intercourse uncomfortable, or even painful. Sometimes this can be due to fungal infection in the vagina, because of reduced immunity caused by chemotherapy. In this case the soreness is often accompanied by itching and irritation, and sometimes a white or yellowish vaginal discharge. If this does happen, then a short course of antifungal drugs will usually clear this up very quickly, in a matter of a few days. So if you do suspect this problem, do mention it to your nurses or doctors. Vaginal dryness often develops during treatment because of hormonal changes caused by the chemotherapy (these may often be temporary and disappear a few months after treatment is over, but they can be unpleasant at the time). If vaginal dryness is a problem, then there are a number of solutions. There are a variety of lubricants that you can buy at chemists or supermarkets which you and your partner can use; these include KY jelly, Senselle, Sylk and Astroglide; or even simple glycerine can be used as an alternative, although unlike the others it is not water soluble and so is a bit more sticky. Another alternative is Replens, which again can be bought over the counter. This is a gel that is a longer-acting vaginal moisturizer, and if used three times a week it can help to overcome vaginal dryness and irritation.

There are also creams or gels for vaginal use that you can only get on prescription. These contain small amounts of the female hormone oestrogen, which nourishes the lining of the vagina and makes it more moist. These products include Vagifem, Ovestin, Premarin and Ortho-Gynest. So if vaginal discomfort is a problem, do talk to your medical team about it, as there may be a very quick and simple solution.

Men may often find that getting an erection is more difficult while they are having chemotherapy and for some time afterwards. This may have a variety of causes, which may be both emotional and physical. Anxiety and depression can both play a part here, and once again just talking about and understanding the problem may make a difference, and adjusting your love making to a pattern where the man needs more time, encouragement and stimulation than before might make a difference. If depression is a problem, then antidepressants may help. If there is a more physical basis for the difficulty, as a result of either the treatment given or the effects of the cancer itself, then drugs like sildenafil (Viagra) vardenafil (Levitra) or tadalafil (Cialis) may help. These are only available on prescription so you would need to discuss this with your doctor. Other solutions for physical problems include small injections of drugs like papavarine or alprostadil (Caverjet, Viridal), which you can be taught to give as injections directly into the penis, or, in the case of alprostadil, alternatively as pellets inserted into the penis.

Another approach is the use of vacuum pumps, which can be applied to the penis before intercourse to stimulate an erection. Sorting out the right approach to this problem can be difficult and it is something where you probably need to talk to your doctor to get his or her advice on what can be done to help.

As already mentioned, depression can be a cause of loss of interest in sex at this time. Feeling low and miserable at times while you are having chemotherapy is very understandable, but for some people this tips over into clinical depression, which becomes a more constant problem where your mood is low all the time, and nothing and nobody seems to be able to cheer you up, and life just seems pointless and hopeless. A loss of sex drive is almost always part of the picture of clinical depression. If this describes the way you are feeling, then do discuss things with your family doctor or hospital specialist because there are very good drugs that can be given to treat clinical depression, and the benefits can often be rapid and dramatic, so this is not a problem that you should suffer, when such easy, safe and effective help is available.

Another physical factor that may influence your sex life is a change in your physical appearance, or body image. This may be due to treatment you have had before chemotherapy, such as an operation like a mastectomy, where a breast has been removed, or a bowel surgery that has left you with a colostomy, or it may be the presence of a central line needed for your chemotherapy treatment.

Once again, changes in body image affect everyone differently. Some people take them in their stride and feel that a change in their physical appearance has little or nothing to do with the real 'them' and makes little or no difference to the person they are, whereas, at the other extreme, some people feel completely devastated by the change. Similarly, the effect on partners can be very variable, with some feeling that a mere physical change has not altered the person they know and love, while others find the altered appearance more unsettling.

Talking is the key to adjusting to this situation. The likelihood is that if you are worried, your partner will be able to offer you reassurance that 'you' are still the person they love and care for and that any change in your appearance makes no difference to those feelings.

In terms of physical intimacy, you or your partner might at first find that change offputting. The probability is that after talking about it, that feeling would lessen or disappear. But if it remains a tension, then it might be possible to get round it by adjusting the technique of your love making so that you could hide the change, covering the area, or keeping certain bits of clothing on during intercourse. Sometimes these new ways of love making actually lead not only to a renewal of desire, but an increase in enjoyment with the novelty of the new approaches to sex.

This section has tended to look at the problem relating to sexuality during and after chemotherapy. But although there will always be times when sex does not appeal, many people find that they can continue not only to have sex during the time of their treatment, but to carry on enjoying it. And if you feel like it, then there is no reason at all why you should not go ahead and have some fun!

Friends and neighbours

Having cancer, and having chemotherapy, can sometimes alter day-to-day relationships with friends and neighbours. On occasions, the changes can be for the better, sometimes for the worse. If there is a problem, then it usually comes down to communication, with either them not understanding your feelings, or you not understanding theirs.

Everyone handles their cancer, and its treatment, differently. You may feel most comfortable by trying to keep things as much to yourself as possible, not sharing your thoughts and feelings with other people, carrying on as near normal as possible. If this is a positive way forward for you, if it helps you feel empowered and in control of your situation, and makes you feel stronger, then that is fine. But if you are simply trying to put a brave face on things because you don't want to burden other people, feeling that if you do so you will be letting yourself down or giving in, then think again because so often sharing your worries and talking things through can be very helpful and supportive. Bringing anxieties and stresses into the open can make them seem far less troubling than bottling them up.

Similarly, friends and neighbours may feel uncertain about how to handle your situation. Should they rush in with offers of help? Should they ask you about how you are getting on, or should they avoid the subject and pretend nothing is happening? They may worry that visiting you will make you tired, or expose you to the risk of minor infections. They may even worry that they could 'catch' cancer from you (which, of course, can never happen).

There are many ways of coping, and it is down to you how you decide to handle this situation. If you want to try and carry on as normally as possible, and feel you cope best in that way, then let people know. Equally, if you are happy to talk about what is happening to you, and if by sharing some, or all, of what you are going through makes life easier, then again let those around you know that you would welcome their questions and concerns. Or you may just want the practical support they can give: help with the shopping, lifts to and from the hospital, looking after the children once in a while, without the emotional involvement of talking about your thoughts and feelings. But however you want to deal with things, it will make life easier for them – and, more importantly, for you – if you let them know.

Telling them might be something you find quite straightforward, or you might feel it is difficult and that it is just one more burden to deal with. If this is the case, then getting your partner, or someone close to you in the family, to have a word with friends and neighbours for you could solve the problem.

9

Clinical trials

Cancer chemotherapy has made enormous progress over the last 50 to 60 years. Most of that progress has been due to developments in traditional chemotherapy drugs – that is, cytotoxic treatment – with the discovery of new drugs and a better understanding of the way to use them. In breast cancer and prostate cancer, however, improvements in hormonal treatments have also made an important contribution. As a result of these changes, many more people are cured of their cancers than previously, and the cure rate continues to improve every year. Furthermore, as a result of the improvements in drug treatment for their particular illness, countless people who have incurable cancer will now live much longer than could ever have been believed possible in the 1950s and 1960s.

New chemotherapy drugs are still appearing, and new combinations of existing drugs are being tested. In addition to this, we now have whole new families of drugs becoming available for cancer treatment with agents like monoclonal antibodies, such as trastuzumab (Herceptin) and bevacuzimab (Avastin), and chemicals like imatinib (Glivec) and gefitinib (Iressa). These developments are exciting and they promise much for the future.

But a word of caution may not be out of place here. It seems that almost every week there is a newspaper report, a magazine article or a television story about some new major breakthrough in the drug treatment of cancer, with a novel compound producing wonderful results. However, many of these offer the illusion of future hope, rather than the reality of proven results. They often deal with the earliest stages of testing of a new drug, frequently when it has only been used in the laboratory and not on any patients at all, and then use these findings as the basis for all the excitement. Eager researchers, pharmaceutical companies with a vested interest, and even cancer charities anxious to attract publicity and donations, will often encourage the media, who are always keen for stories, since cancer 'sells' and, before you know it, the gleam in a laboratory scientist's eye has become the new 'magic bullet' for cancer.

All too often, anxious patients and concerned relatives and friends hear these reports and believe that if they cannot get this new drug then they must be missing out – in other words, feel that their chances of a cure, or an increase in life expectancy, are being jeopardised – when in reality there may be little or no evidence that the compound has any effect at all. At the same time, this pursuit of new, highly publicized treatments can often blind people to the fact that very active, good, tried and tested therapies already exist for their particular type of cancer, which can offer them an excellent chance of successful treatment.

So novelty is not everything. There is already a huge range of treatments that have proved their worth, and that are all freely available on the NHS for people with cancer.

Why do we need trials?

These days many people who are going to have chemotherapy will be offered the chance to take part in a clinical trial. The thought of being in a trial can often be quite worrying, with the fear that you might be a guinea pig for the researches of some mad scientist. But clinical trials are vital to the progress of cancer treatment, and nowadays there are so many safeguards for patients that you need not have any real anxieties.

Fifty years ago there were virtually no clinical trials. Doctors made their decisions about their patients' treatment based on their training and experience. Often those decisions were easy to make – if someone had appendicitis, then you needed to operate to remove their appendix; if someone had pneumonia, then you needed to give them antibiotics. But as more new treatments began to appear, it became more difficult to be sure which was the best treatment to use in any particular situation. And so clinical trials were developed so that treatments that seemed to be more or less equally effective for a particular condition could be compared to see if one really was any better than the other.

In the 1960s the thalidomide disaster occurred, where women were given that drug during early pregnancy to treat morning sickness. It was only later discovered that in many cases thalidomide caused damage to the growing embryo, leading to severe deformities of the limbs. This led to new rules about the testing of drugs before they could be used for routine treatment. Before thalidomide there had been very little done to make sure that new drugs were safe when they were brought into use. Since the disaster of thalidomide, all new drugs have to go through careful trials or studies to make sure that their possible side effects are fully understood, and that they can be used safely.

This means that there are broadly two types of clinical trial: those that are used in the early stages of a drug's development, to test its safety and effectiveness, and those that are used to compare new treatments, once they have proved to be safe and effective, to see if they offer any advantage over existing treatments. The early trials are often called Phase 1 and Phase 2 trials, whereas the comparisons of treatments are called Phase 3 trials.

Most people who have cancer and are offered trial entry will be asked if they would like to take part in Phase 3 studies. Usually only people who have very advanced cancer, and who are no longer likely to benefit from more established treatments, will be offered entry into the more experimental Phase 1 and 2 studies, where the value of the new treatment, and its possible side effects, are still uncertain.

Comparative (Phase 3) clinical trials

Almost every week, the newspapers report some new wonder drug for cancer treatment. These stories usually end with a sentence or two explaining that the results are at an early stage and that more testing will need to be done before the drug can be widely used. Unfortunately, the great majority of these 'wonder drugs' fail to pass the assessments of Phase 1 and 2 trials, either proving ineffective or showing unacceptable toxicity. For the tiny handful of compounds that do successfully overcome these hurdles, the final test is the Phase 3 comparison with the best of the currently available treatments.

There is a tendency to think that just because something is new, it will be better. But for many types of cancer there are well-established, and very effective, therapies. So any new drug must show it has something to add to these older drugs, either by being better at treating the cancer, or being just as good but having fewer side effects, or offering some other benefit.

Phase 3 cancer clinical trials are carefully designed by teams of oncologists and statisticians. They produce a protocol, a document that sets out exactly what the trial is trying to discover, and how it will be carried out. These protocols then have to be approved by panels of experts who look at the scientific value of the work, and an Ethics Committee, which includes lay members, to ensure that the study is safe and the well-being of people who take part in it is protected. So any Phase 3 trial will have been very carefully checked before it is allowed to go ahead.

Usually these trials will compare two or more different treatments for a particular type and stage of cancer. If doctors already had good evidence that one of these treatments is better than the others, they would not need to do the study. These trials are done when the available results suggest that treatments are quite similar, and more careful testing is needed to see if one really is better than the others.

Sometimes a new treatment may become available for a condition where there was no treatment on offer in the past. In this situation, if the merits of the new treatment are still not certain, a trial may be done where it is compared with an inactive compound, or placebo. In this way, one group of people in the study will have a harmless but completely ineffective drug, which would be the same as the old situation of having no treatment, and the results will be compared with those of the others in the trial who are getting the new active drug.

Most trials are designed in such a way that if a particular treatment clearly shows a benefit over the other treatments being tested, then the study can be stopped, and everyone offered the most effective drug.

Nearly all of these comparative Phase 3 trials will be randomized. This means that when someone goes into the study they will have the various treatment options explained to them, but neither they, nor their doctors, will be able to choose which treatment they have. This choice will usually be made by a telephone call to the Trial Centre, where the treatment will be allocated, according to a pattern predetermined by a computer. The reason for this is that if people were left to choose the treatment they preferred, or accept recommendations from their doctors, this could influence the results of the study and lead to bias in favour of a particular treatment, which would in turn lead to false results. So if you have already made up your mind what treatment you really want, then taking part in a trial is probably not for you as the final decision on what will be done is taken out of your hands.

If you are invited to take part in a clinical trial, a number of things should happen, including:

- Your doctor should give you a full explanation of what is involved. This will often be backed up by a talk with a research doctor or nurse involved in running the study.
- You should receive written information in the form of a 'patient information sheet', giving you details of the study and what it will mean for you.
- You should be given time to think about whether or not you want to take part, and should never be asked to make an instant decision.
- You should be given the chance to ask any questions you have about the study.
- No one should ever put pressure on you to try and make you join a trial.

Often, taking part in a trial will mean that you have more hospital visits for check-ups and tests than normal. This is because of the various things that are being measured in the study and the need for very careful monitoring of how you are progressing. Some people like this, and are glad of the extra care and attention involved, while others might find it inconvenient to have more appointments and investigations than is usually necessary. Once again, it pays to make sure you know what will be involved before you make a decision as to whether or not to take part.

If you are offered the chance to take part in a trial and decide not to, this should not affect your future treatment, or in any way affect the care and attention you receive from your doctors and nurses. They will respect your decision and will still continue to try and give you the best possible treatment and look after you just as well as if you were in the trial.

Overall, about one in ten people who have cancer will take part in a clinical trial at some time during their treatment, and most of these will be trials of different types of chemotherapy. For the last 40 years, clinical trials have been the cornerstone for the improvement in the results of treatment with chemotherapy. There are many landmark studies that have resulted in better cure rates for numerous different types of cancer, or years of extra life for people with advanced, incurable tumours, and many others that have brought improvements to people's quality of life by reducing the side effects of treatment.

10

How do you know if treatment has worked?

When you have finished your chemotherapy, and recovered from any side effects, it is natural to want to know whether the treatment has worked. However, it can be very difficult, if not impossible, to know this for sure.

Generally, chemotherapy is given in one of two situations in cancer treatment. It may be used after a primary cancer has been removed by surgery, in order to reduce the risk of the cancer coming back or spreading to other parts of the body. This is adjuvant therapy. Chemotherapy may also be used when the cancer is too widespread, or too advanced for treatment with surgery or radiotherapy. In this situation, it may still be possible to achieve a cure, but often the aim is to control the cancer, leading to an increase in life expectancy and relief of any unpleasant symptoms, rather than being able to get rid of it completely.

Adjuvant therapy

If you have adjuvant chemotherapy, all detectable traces of your cancer will already have been removed by an operation, or radiotherapy, or a combination of these treatments. The reason for giving cytotoxic drugs is because your doctors feel there is a risk that you might still have microscopic traces of cancer in your body, which, over a period of months or years, would grow. This might lead to the growth coming back at its original site (this is called a local recurrence) or to seedlings of tumour appearing in other places (giving rise to secondary cancers, also known as metastases).

In this situation, there is no way of knowing for certain whether or not there are still any cancer cells in your body. Doing x-rays, or scans, or blood tests doesn't help because any remaining tiny seedlings of cancer (which may still contain millions of cancer cells) will be too small to show up on these tests. So what is being treated is the risk that you might have cancer cells left behind, and giving chemotherapy will increase your chances of a complete, permanent, cure.

This means that although many people who have adjuvant chemotherapy will still have traces of cancer, many others will not, and will actually be having the chemotherapy unnecessarily because they are already cured – but unfortunately there is no way of telling who really does, or does not, still have cancer.

Also, although many people who have cancer still present, and who have chemotherapy, will go on to be cured as a result of the treatment, for others the chemotherapy will not work, because their cancer cells are resistant to the drugs, and eventually their cancer will come back. So having adjuvant chemotherapy doesn't guarantee a cure, but it does improve your chances of a successful outcome.

Because there is nothing to measure at the beginning of adjuvant therapy, this means that there will be nothing to measure at the end of treatment. So there is absolutely no way of knowing if the treatment has worked. Since all the scans, x-rays and blood tests that were done would have been normal before your chemotherapy was given, checking them again afterwards will not tell you anything about how well the treatment has worked.

Unfortunately, with adjuvant therapy, only time will tell if the treatment has been successful. Depending on the type of cancer you have had, if between five to ten years later you are still well and with no sign of cancer, then you can be sure that the treatment has worked. This uncertainty can be difficult to live with, but you can take the consolation that by having the treatment you will have done everything possible to get rid of the cancer, and that the likelihood of a cure is greater than if you had not had the chemotherapy.

Although nobody can ever be certain, your oncologist ought to be able to give you an idea of the chances of success of the treatment. For example, they may say that if you just had an operation to remove the cancer and no further treatment, then your chance of a cure would be about 60 per cent, and by having adjuvant chemotherapy you have increased that chance to 80 per cent. In other words, of every ten people who had surgery only, six would be cured, but of every ten people who had surgery and chemotherapy, eight would be cured. So having the chemotherapy will have made a cure much more likely, but it still does not guarantee that things will be all right as there is still a two out of ten chance that the cancer could come back. The exact figures will obviously vary from person to person, and from cancer to cancer, but it is usually possible to give this sort of forecast. Armed with this information, you can then decide whether you think it is worthwhile to have the treatment in the first place, and also get an idea of how likely it is to be successful.

More widespread or more advanced cancer

In this situation there are a number of different ways in which the success of chemotherapy can be gauged.

If a cancer is more widespread, then it is quite likely that it will be causing symptoms. The sort of symptoms that occur vary with the type of cancer and the parts of the body that are affected. Common symptoms include tiredness, pain, breathlessness, loss of appetite (often with some weight loss) and sickness (nausea and vomiting). If chemotherapy eases these symptoms, and makes you feel better, then this is encouraging and suggests that the treatment is working.

Although relief from upsetting symptoms is very worthwhile, it is something that is quite difficult to measure precisely. So although your doctors will be very pleased to see any improvement in how you are feeling, they will be anxious to look for other signs to make sure the treatment is working. This usually means finding something they can measure. This may be a tumour lump that can actually be felt, or an area, or areas, of cancer showing up on scans or x-rays. These can be measured before you start treatment, and those measurements can then be checked at regular intervals during your treatment to make sure things are going well.

Several things may happen as a result of chemotherapy. It may be that a cancer that was growing before you started treatment no longer increases in size, and stays very much the same. This is known as stable disease, or disease stabilization – the cancer is not growing, but neither is it getting any smaller. If the tumour actually begins to shrink in size, then it is called a remission, or a response. If the growth reduces to half its original size, or less, this is called a partial remission, or partial response. Sometimes the chemotherapy will result in all signs of the cancer disappearing – there will no longer be anything to see or feel, and scans, x-rays and blood tests will all go back to normal. When this happens, it is known as a complete remission, or a complete response.

When a complete remission occurs, this is not necessarily the same as a cure. As we saw when we were looking at adjuvant therapy, it is still possible for there to be tiny traces of cancer present in the body even when all the tests are normal, and these could grow back at a future date to cause a relapse, with a return of the cancer.

When a complete remission does occur, the chances of this translating into a permanent cure depend on the type of cancer you have had, and how extensive it was when treatment started. So your specialist will often be able to give you an idea of whether a complete remission is likely to be temporary, or whether a permanent cure might be possible. Even if your doctors think a cure might be on the cards, they will not be able to say this for certain, and once again the only way of knowing for sure is the passage of time.

Epilogue

What next?

You have reached the end of your treatment. It's over. The last blood test has been checked, the last drip has run through, you've swallowed your last anti-sickness tablet. You've made it. A huge sigh of relief. And then . . .

For many people, finishing chemotherapy can be a surprisingly difficult time. Certainly, there are no more of the frequent trips to hospital, no more tests, no more drugs, and no more side effects. But for the last few months, all those sessions have provided a routine, a structure to life. And they have meant that you had got to know the nurses and doctors, and other members of the team, who were looking after you. You had regular support, regular check-ups, and people to talk to about problems and concerns.

Now you are on your own, and that can be hard.

You probably don't feel quite as well as you had expected. The sickness may have stopped, your hair may be growing back, other things may be settling down, but you are likely to still feel pretty tired, and may be wondering how long that weariness will take to disappear.

You've got your next appointment with the specialist, in a month or so, but that leaves a lot of time for you to wonder how things have gone, how successful your treatment has been, and what the future holds. A whole range of thoughts, feelings and emotions that have been shelved or suppressed during the hurly-burly of treatment can now surface, and may take you by surprise.

So be prepared for this to be a more difficult time than you had thought during all those weeks or months when you just couldn't wait for the day when it would all be over.

Half the battle in coping with this period is to realize that you might not find it as easy as you had expected. Be ready for the feelings of loss of contact with the hospital team, and friends you had made during your time on treatment; be ready for the fact that, although the acutely upsetting side effects of treatment are over, there is still a background weariness that limits how much you can do; be prepared for the questions and uncertainties about the future that will come crowding into your mind.

If you are lucky enough to have supportive, understanding family and friends, then this time will be easier. Chatting things through with people, who may do no more than just listen, can be very helpful. If you are on your own, then it may be more difficult, but planning and enjoying a holiday, or days out, or even just local visits and shopping trips can all provide a distraction and help fill the gap in life left by the end of your treatment.

If you are having difficulty coming to terms with your feelings at this time, or if you are feeling very low and unable to talk to those close to you, it might be a good idea if you have a chat with your specialist nurse or GP. They might suggest some form of counselling, which can be very helpful in this situation, or it may be that you have actually become clinically depressed, and a course of antidepressants might transform things for you.

For many people this becomes quite a spiritual period, not necessarily with a turn to conventional religion, but still a time for personal reflection about life.

Being diagnosed with cancer, and going through a major treatment like chemotherapy because of that diagnosis, brings people face to face with questions of life and death. For many people it is a time to take stock of their life, and its meaning. A time to look at where you want life to go in the future. A time to work out what is important to you.

You are likely to look back on your diagnosis, and treatment. To wonder why it was you who got the cancer. You may feel, whatever your doctors and nurses have told you, that there were things in your life that contributed to you getting the illness, things that you want to change in the future. And your treatment, if it involved chemotherapy, will almost certainly have been a major event in life. Some of that experience will have been positive, and some undoubtedly will have been negative, but you have come through it. You will in some ways be a different person, you will have faced up to and taken on challenges, handled situations you had never expected to meet and, one way or another, worked your way through them. Making sense of it all will take time, but you will have learnt a lot about yourself, and usually the insights that come from this are positive, realizing that you can, that you did, deal with a situation that most people think of as a terrifying ordeal. You are likely to be emotionally stronger, with a justifiable pride in your achievement as a survivor of it all.

Your body may have been battered and drained by the therapies you have gone through, your mind may still be reeling to cope with all the changes in your life and how to make sense of the future. You may feel that the whole experience has enriched your life, or you may feel confused, uncertain and even bitter that fate gave you the cancer in the first place. But the fact that you have worked your way through the trauma of being told you have cancer, and then journeyed through months of treatment, with all its demands and downsides, means that you have survived, you have coped. In fact, you are really pretty amazing, and can look back with justifiable pride on your progress, and take strength from your achievement to build for the future.

Useful addresses

Information about cancer, treatment for cancer, and living with cancer

There are many organizations that offer help and advice to people with cancer, and a lot of these cover just one particular type of cancer. The short list that follows gives details of the main providers of information, and they all give details of, and have links to, many other sources of help that you may find useful.

These organizations will also give you more ideas for further reading – many of them have regularly-updated lists of books, booklets and other reading material.

Cancer Research UK
PO Box 123
Lincoln's Inn Fields
London WC2A 3PX
Tel: 020 7121 6699
www.cancerhelp.org.uk

As well as funding research on cancer, this organization has a website that gives information about different types of cancer, and their treatment, as well as a comprehensive list of clinical trials currently in progress.

CancerBACUP
3 Bath Place
Rivington Street
London ECA 3JR
Tel: 0808 800 1234
www.cancerbacup.org.uk

CancerBACUP is a comprehensive information service for patients. It offers a telephone helpline to specially trained cancer nurses, who can give advice on all aspects of cancer and its treatment. It also produces nearly 70 booklets, and more than 200 factsheets on all aspects of cancer. There are also more than 1,000 questions and answers about cancer on its website (the website also has the texts of all the booklets and factsheets, and links to many other useful organizations).

Macmillan Cancer Relief
89 Albert Embankment
London SE1 7UQ
Tel: 0808 808 2020
www.macmillan.org.uk

In addition to funding cancer nursing services, this organization provides a number of publications on cancer, including a useful booklet on benefits and financial help for cancer patients (all listed on the website). The website also has useful information on various aspects of cancer, including a directory of local cancer support groups, and patients' stories about cancer.

DIPEx
www.dipex.org

The initials stand for 'Database of individual patient experiences'. The website covers a number of different illnesses, but has an extensive section on cancer. This not only gives some background information on various types of cancer, but has lots of stories from people who have had cancer, and gone through chemotherapy.

Other information and advice

Benefits Enquiry Line for People with Disabilities
Tel: 0800 882200
www.dwp.gov.uk

This is a national helpline that gives information about the benefits that are available for people with disabilities (including cancer patients), and their carers.

Citizens Advice Bureaux
www.citizensadvice.org.uk

The Citizens Advice Bureau Service offers free, confidential, advice on a variety of problems that people with cancer might face, like difficulties over money, housing or work. The address of your local office will be in the phone book, and is also on the website.

Index

97